ATRIAL
FIBRILLATION
explained

Dr Warrick Bishop
with Penelope Edman

Thank You For Buying This Book!

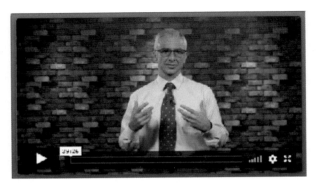

As a special thank you for buying this book, you can get access to our bonus videos and extra information from the website link below.

https://www.healthyheartnetwork.com/afbookbonus

ATRIAL
FIBRILLATION
explained

Understanding the Next Cardiac Epidemic

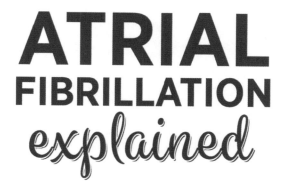

This book is for you, if you

- have atrial fibrillation or know someone who does
- want to understand the condition
- believe that understanding assists with better management
- need to know that you are not alone
- want to know what's going on with your heart
- come from a family with 'bad' hearts
- would enjoy an informative read about a very common condition
- are a doctor wanting a straight-forward refresher or a book you can recommend to your patients

This book is also for you, if you have a heart.

Publisher's Note

The author and editors of this publication have made every effort to provide information that is accurate and complete as of the date of publication. Readers are advised not to rely on the information provided without consulting their own medical advisers. It is the responsibility of the reader's treating physician or specialist, who relies on experience and knowledge about the patient, to determine the condition of, and the best treatment for, the reader. The information contained in this publication is provided without warranty of any kind. The author and editors disclaim responsibility for any errors, mis-statements, typographical errors or omissions in this publication.

National Library of Australia Cataloguing-in-Publication entry

Author:	Dr Warrick Bishop
With:	Penelope Edman, *PAGE 56*
Title:	Atrial Fibrillation Explained
ISBN-13:	978-1-68454-424-0 (Paperback)
ISBN-13:	978-1-68454-425-7 (Hardcover)
ISBN-13:	978-1-097246-595 (Amazon Paperback)
ASIN:	B07RD653D6
Subject:	Cardiac health care
Publisher:	Dr Warrick Bishop
Website:	www.drwarrickbishop.com
Designer:	Cathy McAuliffe, *Cathy McAuliffe Design*
Illustrator:	Cathy McAuliffe, *Cathy McAuliffe Design*

Dedicated to
Mercia,
for the good times

Contents

HOW: TREATMENT

HOW: CONVERSATIONS

WHERE: THE FUTURE

Foreword

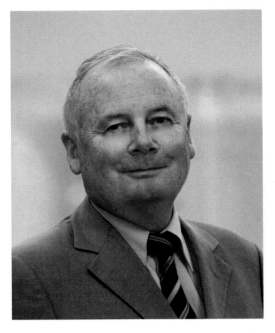

Atrial fibrillation is another of the many medical conditions generally referred to by initials, in this case AF. It is important because it is already common but becoming increasingly so in the face of an ageing community, with more people living with heart disease or the lifestyle and other factors that make AF more likely, such as obesity, sedentary lifestyle, hypertension or diabetes.

AF is an irregular heartbeat and one cause of palpitations. If the heart beats too fast it can cause breathlessness. AF can come and go out of the blue or it can become established and permanent. Many people, though, live their lives with AF without knowing about it.

Unfortunately, that is not all there is to AF. It puts people at higher risk of stroke. One-quarter to one-third of strokes are due to clots formed in the heart in someone with AF. The clot breaks off and causes a blockage in the blood flow to the brain.

This risk can be substantially reduced with modern therapy.

To receive this benefit, people need to know that they have AF and then what they should do. AF requires a team effort involving the people who suffer from AF and their families, their doctors and other health professionals. There can be a number of options for treatment and people need to work with their doctors to agree on what is best for them.

Recently, the Heart Foundation and Cardiac Society of Australia issued their first guidelines on AF for health professionals. This comprehensive document informs health professionals about the latest evidence to guide best practice management of the condition. Doctors, therefore, have access to the best evidence and the latest information, but what about the rest of the community? We know from surveys that knowledge about heart disease in the general community is low.

This book is one of a series written by Dr Warrick Bishop to help remedy the situation. It is a personal account from a busy cardiologist trying to span the gap between what doctors know about AF and what those with AF and their loved ones need to know. It is informed by the latest guidelines but also includes personal anecdotes and the stories of real people who have experienced AF.

The evidence will change as this is an active area of research; new treatments and devices will no doubt come along. However, this book, along with other material produced by the Heart Foundation and other authoritative bodies, will make the reader more informed and better able to avoid AF and its complications.

PROF. GARRY JENNINGS AO

Cardiologist

Executive Director, Sydney Health Partners

Sydney, Australia

Professor Garry Jennings AO is Executive Director of Sydney Health Partners and is recognised as a world leader in translating research into better health outcomes for the community. He is former head of the Baker Heart and Diabetes Institute, and of the Department of Cardiology at The Alfred Hospital in Melbourne. He has had a long association with the Heart Foundation in various leadership roles.

A distinguished cardiologist and researcher, Prof. Jennings has written more than 450 scientific and medical publications, and a number of books on heart disease for the general community.

Preface

Atrial fibrillation is the most common cardiac arrhythmia and untreated or under-treated atrial fibrillation is a major cause of stroke, heart failure, hospitalisations and even death. In many people, atrial fibrillation can cause significant symptoms but in others it can be present with no symptoms.

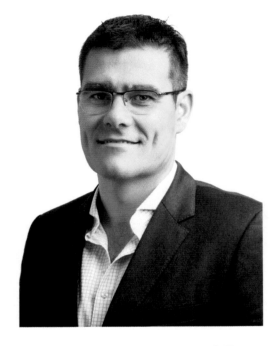

This book provides an excellent introduction to atrial fibrillation and a comprehensive review of the management options available for AF.

The management of atrial fibrillation is complex and can be confusing. A number of different approaches and a number of different strategies are possible, depending on the specifics of the person with atrial fibrillation and the expertise and interest of the treating doctor.

I think this book is an ideal resource for anyone diagnosed with atrial fibrillation or living with someone diagnosed with atrial fibrillation. Presenting to your treating cardiologist or electrophysiologist with a better understanding of atrial fibrillation will improve the doctor-patient experience and ensure that the best outcomes can be achieved.

I have known Dr Warrick Bishop for many years, and we have shared and successfully managed many patients with atrial fibrillation. He is respected and admired by all the patients we have in common.

Warrick has an unique ability to demystify complex medical issues. His style is factually accurate and scientifically complete, yet free of the medical jargon typically used by many in our profession. I have frequently recommended his previous book, *Have You Planned Your Heart Attack?* I also have links to his *Healthy Heart Network* TV show and his podcasts on my office computer.

This is the best patient-focused atrial fibrillation book that I have read.

DR DAVID O'DONNELL

Electrophysiologist and Cardiologist

Director, GenesisCare
Head of Electrophysiology, Austin Hospital

Melbourne, Australia

Dr David O'Donnell is the Chairman of GenesisCare Cardiology, Victoria, and the Board Director for the GenesisCare Network. He is the Head of Electrophysiology at the Austin Hospital, Melbourne, Australia.

Having studied at Melbourne University and the Austin Hospital, his advanced training was in Europe. This led to a clinical focus on ablation for atrial fibrillation and a research interest in the device management of heart failure.

Dr O'Donnell has had a longstanding clinical interest in the management of all aspects of atrial fibrillation. He is one of Australia's most experienced atrial fibrillation ablation specialists, having personally performed more than 3000 procedures. At the same time, he has a specific focus on the lifestyle measures that contribute to AF and the importance of a multi-disciplinary approach to the optimal management of these.

He also has a specific interest in the management of arrhythmias in athletes and currently works with a number of sporting bodies and elite athletes.

Acknowledgements

Atrial Fibrillation Explained has been informed by

2016 ESC Guidelines for the management of atrial fibrillation developed in collaboration with EACTS

Paulus Kirchhof, Stefano Benussi, Dipak Kotecha, Anders Ahlsson, Dan Atar, Barbara Casadei, Manuel Castella, Hans-Christoph Diener, Hein Heidbuchel, Jeroen Hendriks, Gerhard Hindricks, Antonis S Manolis, Jonas Oldgren, Bogdan Alexandru Popescu, Ulrich Schotten, Bart Van Putte, Panagiotis Vardas, ESC Scientific Document Group

Published in the *European Heart Journal*, Volume 37, Issue 38, 7 October 2016, Pages 2893–2962

National Heart Foundation of Australia and the Cardiac Society of Australia and New Zealand: Australian Clinical Guidelines for the Diagnosis and Management of Atrial Fibrillation 2018

NHFA CSANZ Atrial Fibrillation Guideline Working Group, David Brieger, MBBS, PhD, John Amerena, MBBS, FRACP, FCSANZ, John Attia, MD, PhD, FRACP, Beata Bajorek, BPharm, PhD, Kim H. Chan, MBBS, PhD, FRACP, Cia Connell, BPharm, GCPharmPrac, MClinPharm, Ben Freedman, MBBS, PhD, FRACP, Caleb Ferguson, RN Ph, Tanya Hall, Haris Haqqani, MBBS, PhD, FRACP, Jeroen Hendriks, MSc, PhD, Charlotte Hespe, MBBS, DCH, FRACGP, Joseph Hung, MBBS, FRACP, FCSANZ, Jonathan M. Kalman, MBBS, PhD, Prashanthan Sanders, MBBS, PhD, FRACP, John Worthington, MBBS, BSc(Med), FRACP, Tristan D. Yan, MD, MS, PhD, Nicholas Zwar, MBBS, MPH, PhD

Published in *Heart Lung and Circulation*, October 2018 Volume 27, Issue 10, Pages 1209–1266

2019 AHA/ACC/HRS Focused Update of the 2014 HA/ACC/HRS Guideline for the Management of Patients With Atrial Fibrillation: A Report of the American College of Cardiology/American Heart Association Task Force on Clinical Practice Guidelines and the Heart Rhythm Society

January CT, Wann LS, Calkins H, Chen LY, Cigarroa JE, Cleveland Jr JC, Ellinor PT, Ezakowitz MD, Field ME, Furie KL, Heindenreich PA, Murray KT, Shea JB, Tracy CM, Yancey CW. 2019 AHA/ACC/HRS Focused Update of the 2014 HA/ACC/HRS Guideline for the Management of Patients With Atrial Fibrillation, Journal of the American College of Cardiology (2019), doi: https://doi.org/10.1016/j.jacc.2019.01.011

Atrial Fibrillation Explained is not a comprehensive guide to current literature. It is intended to act as a starting point for conversation and further education.

*It is from our hearts
that we lead our lives
and see the world.*

anon.

Introduction -
BEYOND THE GUIDELINES

In 1994, my grandmother, a woman in her 80s, was not in great health. She had been wheelchair-bound for many years because of congenital dislocation of her hips. She had cardiac failure. She had diabetes. She had Paget's disease of bone which affected some of the major bones in her body, including the skull plates of her head. She had cataracts so she couldn't see very well. She had a severe form of rheumatoid arthritis that caused her considerable distress. Then, she was hospitalised and it was found that she had pneumonia. She was a sick woman.

While in hospital, she was diagnosed with a condition called atrial fibrillation. This is an irregular beat of the heart characterised by the loss of the co-ordinated contraction of the top part of the heart, the atrial chambers. The condition affects the pumping capacity of the heart, important because it reduces how well the heart functions as a pump. It can also cause other problems which carry their own risks. One of these is the formation of a clot within the heart which can lead to a stroke.

When this near-blind, wheelchair-bound, 80+ year-old lady with bad rheumatoid arthritis, cardiac failure and diabetes left hospital, because of the atrial fibrillation risk of stroke, she was started on a medication called warfarin.

Warfarin is a blood thinner and works well to reduce the risk of stroke. The problem was that Gran was on multiple tablets already. She couldn't really see what she was doing and so Grandpa looked after her medications. She had a lot of trouble having regular blood tests, a management imperative when using warfarin. Even more importantly, though, because her heart was not working properly, blood was accumulating in her organs. One of the important organs where it was collecting was the liver, and the liver is where warfarin is metabolised or processed.

I saw this as a difficult situation. As high as was the risk of stroke, treatment with warfarin seemed to present a situation that could lead to complications that probably outweighed the benefit, at least for my grandmother. While the medical team had made the decision to commence a blood-thinning agent in keeping with all the guidelines regarding atrial fibrillation, the guidelines didn't consider, specifically, my grandmother's overall medical condition. The guidelines didn't address the needs of a person who was over 80 years of age, visually impaired, a diabetic with rheumatoid arthritis who also had cardiac failure and problems with her liver function, leading to an inability of the body to potentially clear and manage that drug properly and so bring her benefit.

After detailed discussion with her medical team, we thought, on balance, Gran's life was less complicated by using aspirin instead of warfarin. This was not the guideline recommendation but, for her, almost certainly the best and most sensible compromise. She lived at home and then moved to a nursing home where she died about three or four years later, from a stroke.

Atrial fibrillation is a common condition. We know that it affects more than 30 million people worldwide. Statistics show that for adults over 20 years of age, it affects three percent of the population and for adults over 80 years of age, more than 15 percent of the population. So, if you have atrial fibrillation or you know someone who has it, it is no surprise.

Although atrial fibrillation is widespread, the way we manage it shouldn't always be the same for everyone. It is a condition that warrants good information and good education so that patients can be engaged in their own best management. Gran's circumstances highlight that we are all individuals. This requires each patient, maybe also the family but certainly the patient, and the doctor looking at the pros and cons of each intervention and coming to an understanding of the individual's needs and circumstances.

In the following pages, I will explain what the condition is, how we diagnose it, how we manage it and how that impacts on the patient. We will look at the drugs and other approaches that can be involved in treatment. We will scrutinise atrial fibrillation in a way that allows patients and medical practitioners to understand the best way to look after the condition in personal sets of circumstances.

While this book will provide interesting and useful details, it will also pose questions, hopefully resulting in some significant and revealing discussions between you, the individual, and your medical care providers.

Let's begin.

WHAT AND WHO
THE CONDITION

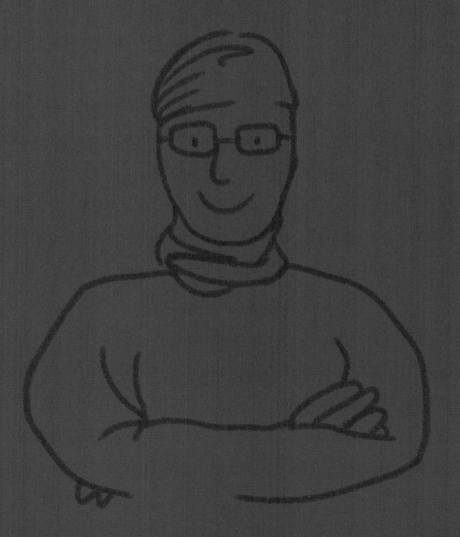

Chapter 1 -
AN OVERVIEW

what is atrial fibrillation?

Atrial fibrillation is a disturbance within the electrical system of the heart which gives rise to a heart rhythm disorder or arrhythmia. This means that the person has an irregular, or abnormal, heartbeat. The term we use to describe it is 'irregularly irregular'. Sudden, rapid, irregular and chaotic heartbeats may be a sign of this common heart rhythm problem. The impact of the condition on the patient ranges from inconvenience to black out, to chest pain and heart failure, with stroke another potential, devastating complication. While atrial fibrillation can be managed, at this time[1] there is no cure.

the heart

The heart is the large muscle that pumps blood through our bodies. The blood supplies nutrients and oxygen, and also removes waste such as carbon dioxide. The heart can be likened to a car engine with compression chambers and valves, an electrical system and a set of fuel lines. It is the **electrical system** which will concern us primarily in the following pages.

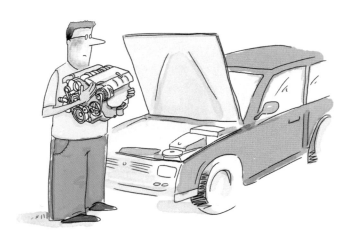

As a car engine has an electrical system for timing, so does the heart. The electrical system in the heart ensures synchronicity and coordinated contraction throughout the heart. It also allows a mechanism for acceleration and deceleration.

The car has pistons and valves as part of its power-generating engine block while the heart has as its pistons the compression chambers, the main one being the ventricle, and valves which stop the blood flowing back from where it came.

To complete our analogy, the car engine also requires a fuel line to supply the engine block. In the human heart, the fuel lines are the coronary arteries that literally provide the life-blood to the engine block, the muscle of the heart.

This muscle, called the myocardium (*myo,* muscle; *cardium,* being of the heart), is a four-chambered structure. There are two chambers on the right-hand side and two chambers on the left-hand side. This means you have **two** pumps, one that accepts the blood back from the body and then pumps it to the lungs, and then a second pump that receives the blood from the lungs and then drives it around the body, the 'right heart' and the 'left heart', respectively. On each side of the heart there is a pre-pumping chamber, the atrium, and a main pumping chamber, the ventricle.

pistons and valves

Blood drains from the body through the veins, collecting into two major veins called the superior vena cava (SVC) and the inferior vena cava (IVC) which drain into the right side of the heart. This oxygen-poor, dark purple, carbon dioxide-rich blood arrives in the right atrium and is given a gentle pump through a one-way valve, the tricuspid valve, into the ventricle which then pumps the blood through another one-way valve, the pulmonary valve, into the pulmonary circulation which takes the blood to the lungs. There, by simple diffusion[2], it is purified and oxygenated; carbon dioxide is released and leaves the body through the breath we exhale, while oxygen, from the air we breathe in, is absorbed.

Bright red, oxygen-rich arterial blood then flows through the four pulmonary veins to the left atrium. The left atrium gives a gentle pump and the blood passes through the mitral valve, another one-way valve, into the left ventricle which then contracts, squeezing blood through the aortic valve into

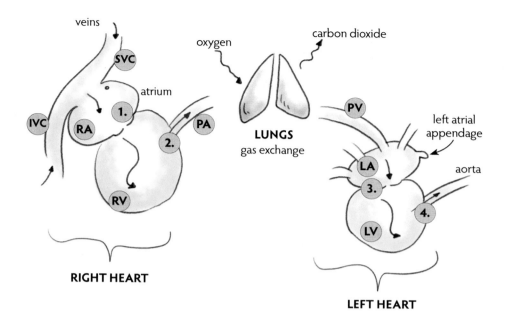

1.	Tricuspid Valve	**PA**	Pulmonary Artery (blood to lungs)
2.	Pulmonary Valve	**PV**	Pulmonary Veins (blood from lungs)
3.	Mitral Valve		
4.	Aortic Valve	**RA** **LA**	
IVC	Inferior Vena Cava	Right Atrium, Left Atrium (pre-pumping chambers)	
SVC	Superior Vena Cava	**RV** **LV**	
		Right Ventricle, Left Ventricle (main pumping chambers)	

the main artery of the body, the aorta, to begin its journey around the body. The contraction of the left ventricle makes the blood flow through the arteries and we feel this as our pulse.

fuel lines

The coronary arteries arise from the aorta as it comes from the left ventricle. They are the first branches in the circulation system. These are the fuel lines of the heart engine.

Cardiovascular disease involves heart and blood vessel diseases, and includes stroke. In a population of 25 million people, it affects one in six, or 3.7 million people, and kills one person every 12 minutes. Cardiovascular disease is often the main cause of hospitalisations in Western countries, in a given year. Although this book is about the electrical system, it is not uncommon for the fuel system and the electrical system to show features of wear and tear simultaneously.

Assessing the health of the arteries is the topic of another book I have written, Have You Planned Your Heart Attack?[3]

A CLOSER LOOK

ARTERIES

It is useful to think of the arteries as the fuel lines supplying the cylinders of the car, transporting blood to different territories (pistons) of the heart muscle. This system consists of the right coronary artery and the left main coronary artery. Within one centimetre, the left coronary artery divides into two main arteries: the left anterior descending artery which provides blood to the anterior surface of the heart, that is the surface nearest the chest wall, and the circumflex artery which supplies blood to the back of the heart or the surface of the heart nearest the spine. The right coronary artery supplies the inferior surface of the heart or the surface that is nearest the diaphragm.

The terms 'right dominant' or 'left dominant' can be used in reference to the origin of the artery that supplies blood to the bulk of the inferior surface of the heart. This is generally from the right coronary artery but sometimes the right coronary artery is smaller, and the circumflex is 'dominant', or bigger, supplying the majority of the inferior surface of the heart. This is called 'left dominant'. This becomes important in terms of the amount of the heart that may be affected by a blockage of the artery, the dominant artery providing blood to a larger territory.

The left anterior descending artery supplies blood to the anterior wall of the heart (nearest the chest wall). Most often, the left anterior descending artery is the largest and most important of the three main coronary arteries. It can be 12 to 14 cm long, while only two to five millimetres in diameter. This is little thicker than a pen refill, yet its blockage can be disastrous. A dominant right coronary artery can be approximately the same size and a non-dominant circumflex can be six to eight centimetres long and 1.5 to three millimetres in diameter.

The major arteries are comprised of fewer than 35 cm in total length and fewer than five millimetres in diameter at their largest.

This is a very vulnerable system.

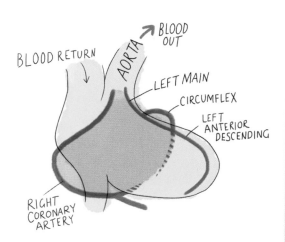

a schematic showing how the blood vessels wrap around the heart

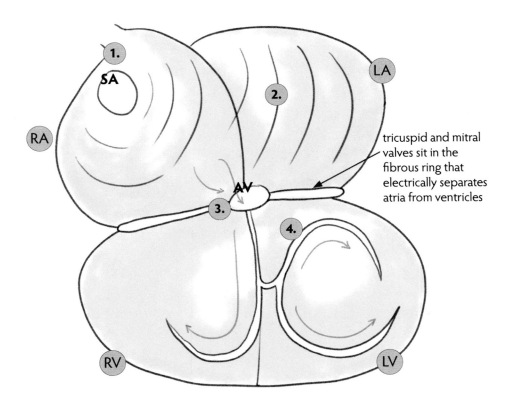

tricuspid and mitral valves sit in the fibrous ring that electrically separates atria from ventricles

1. electrical impulse originates in SA (sinoatrial) node

2. impulse propagates through atria

3. impulse passes through AV (atrioventricular) node

4. impulse is 'delivered' to ventricles through Purkinje fibres (similar to copper wires in the heart)

the electrical system

electrical system coordinates powerful pump

A healthy heart is a highly efficient pump coordinated by its **electrical system**. The atria and ventricles work together, alternately contracting and relaxing, to pump blood through the heart and into the body. The heartbeat is triggered by electrical impulses. The heart pumps three to four litres of blood every minute, with the healthy heart rate between 50 and 100 beats per minute.

Normally, the contractions of the atria are set off by the heart's natural pacemaker, a small area of the heart called the **sinoatrial (SA) node**, located in the top of the right atrium. This is where the electrical activity 'beats the drum' to which the rest of the heart 'marches'.

Electrical impulses travel rapidly throughout the atria, a bit like a Mexican wave, causing the muscle fibres to contract, squeezing blood into the ventricles. To get to the ventricles, these electrical impulses pass through the **atrioventricular (AV) node**, a cluster of cells in the centre of the heart, between the atria and the ventricles. This node acts as a gatekeeper. Passing through this node slows the electrical impulses before they enter the ventricles, thus giving the atria time to contract before the ventricles then contract. Once in the ventricles, the electrical impulse is carried via special cells, Purkinje fibres, that act like wires delivering the signal to the apex of the heart, ensuring that blood is expelled from the furthest point first.

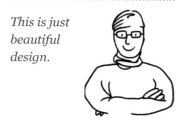

This is just beautiful design.

This normal heart rhythm is known as **sinus rhythm** because it is controlled by the sinoatrial, or sinus, node. In a healthy heart, this beating occurs in a synchronistic and smooth manner. Visualise, if you can, a squid moving through the water. Synchronous. Coordinated. Smooth.

break-down

When this synchronicity breaks down, arrhythmia occurs.

One of the most common forms of heart arrhythmia is atrial fibrillation[4] which, according to the European Society of Cardiology (ESC), is one of the major causes of stroke, heart failure, sudden death and cardiovascular disease in the world. The ESC also predicts that its prevalence will rise steeply in coming years[5].

Atrial fibrillation results in chaotic, or irregular, electrical activity leading to the atria not contracting properly. Instead they shake, vibrate, tremor; they fibrillate. Between 20 and 30 percent of all strokes are due to atrial fibrillation[6]. Long-term atrial fibrillation can damage the structure of the heart and sometimes existing heart problems can trigger atrial fibrillation; hence the association with cardiac morbidity and mortality.

classifications

There are two types of atrial fibrillation: the type that the patient feels, called **overt** or **symptomatic** atrial fibrillation, and the type of which the patient is not aware, called **silent** or **asymptomatic** atrial fibrillation.

Atrial fibrillation classification is also referred to in terms of the time the patient is in the abnormal rhythm: **paroxysmal, persistent** or **permanent** atrial fibrillation.

symptoms

In **overt,** or symptomatic, atrial fibrillation, the person is aware when the condition occurs and/or is present. Sufferers will feel palpitations in the chest, an irregularity, a fluttering which they can describe quite clearly. Some will have shortness of breath on exertion, for example while climbing the stairs or carrying the groceries. Others will notice a decrease in their exercise capacity. Because atrial fibrillation can occur very suddenly, and because the heart is not pumping normally, it can also be associated with low blood pressure and patients may present with a collapse.

In **silent,** or asymptomatic, atrial fibrillation, the person does not feel it at all. It is discovered as an incidental finding. This can occur when the person goes to the general practitioner for a check, say, a blood pressure check, and the doctor notices that the person's pulse is irregular, instead of being strong and regular as a normal sinus rhythm beat should be. The irregularity in the pulse could be atrial fibrillation. Three percent of the population over 75 years of age will have AF and not be aware of having the condition.

Occasionally, the possibility of atrial fibrillation being present is indicated by something else.

An unfortunate and common modern situation is in the setting of a stroke. This is when a blood clot has gone from the heart to the brain. This neurological problem can result in localised weakness, difficulty with speech, difficulty with vision and even lead to death. A stroke that lasts momentarily is called a **T**ransient (doesn't last very long) **I**schaemic (lack of blood flow) **A**ttack or TIA. A stroke and TIAs are triggers in which to look for AF as a potential cause.

Large numbers of people today have heart-related devices implanted, pacemakers, in particular. The interrogation of these devices can be as often as every six months or as long as every 12 months. Either way, when these devices are checked, the heart rhythm can be evaluated. So, it is possible to find that people being seen for pacemaker issues may have atrial fibrillation detected incidentally during a check to ensure the device is working properly.

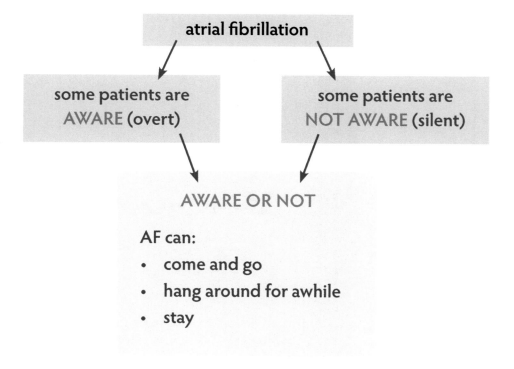

Important to know!

The incidental finding of atrial fibrillation can occur when an ECG (electrocardiogram) is taken.

An example in the hospital where my consulting rooms are located is the pre-operative ECG which is very commonly undertaken for patients over a certain age undergoing procedures with a certain complexity.

It is a really good way to pick up asymptomatic AF, a valuable opportunity to make the diagnosis and initiate appropriate therapy.

A CLOSER LOOK

STROKE

We know stroke is a devastating occurrence. In the simplest terms, stroke is an interruption of the blood flow to the brain, an organ which needs a good supply of blood at all times. If there is any change in that flow, the tissue of the brain can be damaged. Damage to the tissue of the brain from a change in, or interruption to, the blood flow is a stroke.

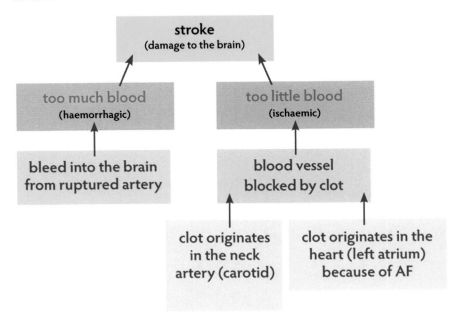

please note that there are other causes of stroke beyond the scope of this discussion

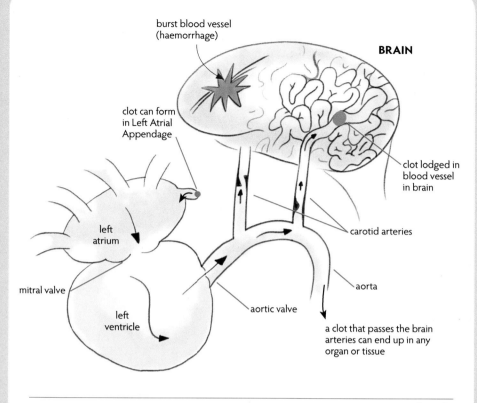

burst blood vessel
(haemorrhage)

BRAIN

clot can form
in Left Atrial
Appendage

clot lodged in
blood vessel
in brain

left
atrium

carotid arteries

mitral valve

aorta

left
ventricle

aortic valve

a clot that passes the brain
arteries can end up in any
organ or tissue

origins of a stroke

There are two main ways a stroke can occur, resulting in an **haemorrhagic** *stroke or an* **ischaemic** *stroke.*

If a blood vessel supplying an area, or territory, in the brain bursts or ruptures, it bleeds into that territory causing damage. This is an **haemorrhagic** *stroke in which too much blood goes into that area of the brain because the artery has been damaged.*

It can be associated with abnormalities of the blood vessels in which there is a thinning and a rupture at that location. It can be related to points of strain within the arteries of the brain when high blood pressure over time causes weakness within the arteries and that can also, with age, lead to situations when blood may rupture from the blood vessel into the tissue of the brain.

Haemorrhagic strokes account for about 15 percent of strokes.

*An **ischaemic** stroke occurs when a clot, also called a thrombus, blocks the artery, leading to a lack of blood flow.*

An ischaemic stroke arises when a clot dislodges from a location within the body and travels to the brain, lodging itself in an artery and thus blocking the artery.

Ischaemic strokes account for the other 85 percent of strokes.

In relation to an ischaemic stroke, there are two main locations where the clot may form. The most common location is within the large blood vessels in the neck, the carotid arteries. A build-up of plaque in these arteries can lead to rupture of that plaque. A clot forms, breaks off, moves to the brain, lodges in one of the blood vessels and stops the blood supply, causing a stroke. Strokes originating in the carotid arteries account for about 50 to 55 percent of ischaemic strokes.

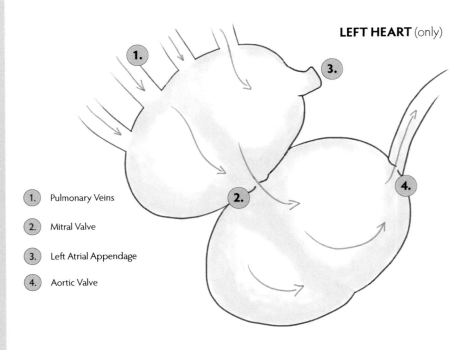

LEFT HEART (only)

1. Pulmonary Veins
2. Mitral Valve
3. Left Atrial Appendage
4. Aortic Valve

LA (Left Atrium) and LAA (Left Atrial Appendage)

In a population of 25 million people, someone has a stroke every 10 minutes, leading to a cost of $5 billion a year.[7]

The other major clot source is the heart as a consequence of atrial fibrillation.

*When the left atrium is not contracting properly, blood can pool within a recess in the left atrium, the **left atrial appendage.** If blood pools in the appendage, a clot can form and subsequently dislodge.*

Such a clot will float into the left atrium, sweep through the mitral valve into the left ventricle. The ventricle will expel blood, including the clot, into the aorta. It will then come to the arch of the aorta where there is an opportunity for that clot to travel to the brain via either of the carotid arteries, and subsequently become lodged in a blood vessel within the brain, leading to an ischaemic stroke.

If the clot passes the brain arteries, it will continue to travel with the blood flow until it finds a place to rest which could be any organ or tissue beyond the brain: the gut, kidneys, liver, spleen or even a toe.

IMPORTANT POINTS A STROKE

A stroke can be

- **haemorrhagic**, bleeding into the brain tissue (about 15 percent)
- **ischaemic**, from reduced blood flow (about 85 percent)
  - from problems within the carotid arteries (50-55 percent)
  - from the atrium (left atrial appendage) as a consequence of atrial fibrillation (about 30 percent)

an incidental finding

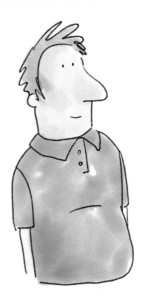

Peter was a 65-year-old man when his atrial fibrillation was found incidentally. A week or so before I met him, late in 2017, Peter was undergoing a routine colonoscopy, a test to look in his lower bowel. The anaesthetist who was looking after him found his pulse to be 'irregularly irregular' with a controlled rate. An ECG and subsequent monitoring confirmed that Peter was in atrial fibrillation, although he had had no clue as to his situation as he had experienced no symptoms. This is not entirely uncommon. A number of people do walk around with silent or asymptomatic fibrillation.

When I spoke with Peter, it turned out that he had seen his GP about three months earlier. His blood pressure and pulse, which were checked at the time, were said to be okay. This suggests that he had gone into fibrillation in that intervening period. Peter's general health also included some hypertension for which he was on therapy and central adiposity or weight around the belly. This can be a marker of prediabetes and is worth keeping in mind. He did not exercise much.

When we looked at Peter's risk of a stroke on the CHA2DS2-VASc score (a clinical predictor for estimating the risk of stroke in patients with atrial fibrillation) he had a score of two: one for age and one for hypertension. I would have added an extra score for prediabetes. However, with a score of two, his risk of stroke was considered mild to moderate with the recommendation that he should be on full anticoagulation.

We also had other information available. A 24-hour heart rate monitor showed that in the asymptomatic state, on average, Peter's heartbeat in atrial fibrillation was nearly 100 beats a minute, going as high as 180 beats a minute at times of exertion. For someone in his mid-60s, that's a very fast heartbeat and I was quite surprised that he was asymptomatic.

An ultrasound of his heart showed that the structure and function of Peter's heart were relatively normal, although his atria were mildly to moderately dilated.

As a result of the CHA2DS2-VASc score, I started Peter on full anticoagulation. I also included in the therapy a drug to try to slow the heartbeat down. A heart that's revving so quickly simply does not fill properly and therefore doesn't pump properly, and so patients almost invariably describe some shortness of breath. This should give him more puff as the heart pumps better.

Another consideration for Peter was whether or not we should attempt to restore sinus rhythm. On occasions, we can be caught between trying to restore normal rhythm and leaving people in atrial fibrillation. The lack of symptoms, as in the case of Peter, can suggest an approach that simply controls the heart rate.

However, in this particular situation, the patient is relatively young. My observation over the years, and there is some research coming through to support this, is that if we restore sinus rhythm we may have a positive effect on any morphological, or structural, change the heart could undergo. What I mean by that is, if we leave people in atrial fibrillation for many years, we see changes in the heart as a consequence of that atrial fibrillation. The most notable alteration is that the atria dilate or enlarge. Another observation, and I have a number of cases in which this has occurred, is the atrioventricular ring that connects the atrium to the ventricle also dilates as the atria dilate. If the AV ring dilates, then the fixtures for the valves that it holds, particularly for the tricuspid valve which is on the right side of the heart, can be stretched. As it stretches, the cusps of that tricuspid valve do not come together as well as they should. So, although I haven't yet[8] attempted to restore sinus rhythm in Peter, it's a serious consideration so that the structure of his heart can be maintained in its best condition for as long as possible.

Regardless of whether I return him to sinus rhythm or not, Peter will be on anticoagulation for the remainder of his life. The CHA2DS2-VASc score is high enough, and with his being completely unaware of symptoms, I wouldn't begin to rely on him to tell me when he's in and out of the rhythm.

time in rhythm

If atrial fibrillation is experienced for a short time, between 24 and 48 hours but no longer than a week, it is called **paroxysmal** atrial fibrillation, meaning that it comes and goes. This classification is characterised by a short period when the patient has the abnormal rhythm and then the heart reverts back to sinus rhythm.

If the abnormal rhythm is present in the patient for longer than seven days, it is called **persistent** (staying there longer) AF.

Permanent (long-standing) atrial fibrillation means it has been present for longer than a year.

What if the patient is asymptomatic?

Deciding whether the atrial fibrillation is paroxysmal, persistent or permanent is almost impossible to ascertain, if this is the case. How do you know when it started? Simply, you don't!

Some clues can be found from other investigations. The simplest hint is the longer a person has been in atrial fibrillation, the greater the likelihood there will be changes in the atria of the heart. Dilation of the atria will be more pronounced the longer the heart has been out of rhythm.

While one of the management strategies is to attempt to return a patient to sinus rhythm, this is not the case for all sufferers of persistent or permanent atrial fibrillation. The clinician will need to decide if the patient's condition is to be accepted long-term, based on factors relevant and specific to that patient. If the decision is to leave the person in atrial fibrillation, then controlling the rate of the heartbeat and management of the risk of clot formation within the heart become the foci.

effective management

Atrial fibrillation is associated with a poorer quality of life for sufferers as symptoms include lethargy, palpitations, breathlessness, chest tightness, sleeping difficulties and psychosocial distress.

AF cannot be cured.

In managing atrial fibrillation, medical carers look to the efficiency of the heart as a pump, its rate and its rhythm, and stroke mitigation as the significant concerns. The condition, regardless of its type and time in arrhythmia, can be managed with medication, lifestyle adjustments and, sometimes, through procedural interventions.

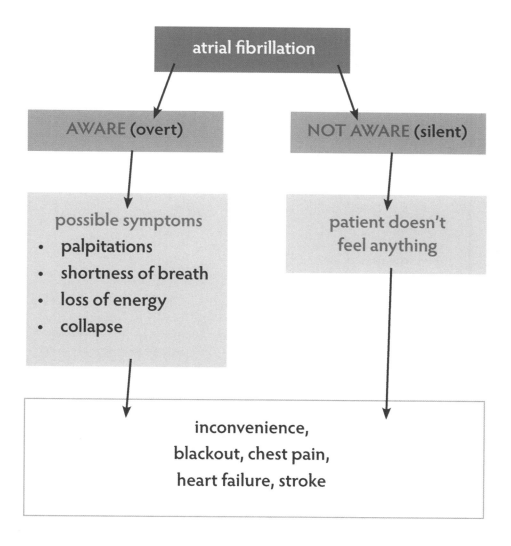

potential outcomes of AF

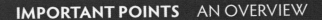

Atrial fibrillation

- is characterised by the loss of coordinated atrial activity so that the person's heartbeat becomes 'irregularly irregular'

- leads to the decreased efficiency of the heart as a pump

- is associated with a significant increased risk of stroke

- can be either overt (with symptoms) or silent (no symptoms)

- can be paradoxical (lasting hours), persistent (lasting days or longer) or permanent (ongoing)

- currently has no cure, but it can be managed

[1]   2019

[2]   The term 'simple diffusion' refers to a process whereby a substance passes through a membrane without the aid of an intermediary. The force that drives the substance from one side of the membrane to the other is the force of diffusion. Types of molecules that can do this include carbon dioxide and oxygen. (http://academic.brooklyn.cuny.edu/biology/bio4fv/page/simple.htm)

[3]   This has been published in the United States as Know Your Real Risk of Heart Attack.

[4]   Other arrhythmia include fast beats, missed beats and extra beats. We touch on these later.

[5]   2016 ESC Guidelines for the management of atrial fibrillation developed in collaboration with EACTS; European Heart Journal (2016) 37. 2893-2962; p. 2899

[6]   ibid; p. 2899

[7]   the Australian Stroke Foundation website

[8]   early 2019

ARE ALL CLOTS THE SAME?

Clotting is a normal function that is required in the body for our existence. Otherwise, if we were to cut ourselves we would bleed to death. There are times, though, when clots can cause problems and threaten our existence.

*A clot which forms in **an artery of the heart**, blocking the artery, can cause a heart attack. Bad.*

*If a clot forms in the **left atrial appendage** of the heart, it can break free and travel to the brain through the arteries which supply blood and oxygen. A block in an artery to the brain causes a stroke. Bad again.*

*If the clot forms in a **carotid artery** and moves to the brain, it can also cause a stroke. Still bad.*

*There are, however, other places in the body where clots can form. Most well-known are the **legs**. A **D**eep **V**ein **T**hrombosis (DVT) can form there due to immobility for a variety of reasons such as a long aeroplane flight or after surgery. If the clot breaks off, it travels back to the heart passing through the right heart and into the lungs causing a very serious medical problem, pulmonary (pertaining to the lungs) thromboembolism (blood clot that moves through the bloodstream). You guessed it. Very bad.*

Problems from blood clotting are treated according to where the clot originated in the body. In particular, clots formed within the coronary arteries (heart attack) and the carotid arteries (ischaemic stroke) are treated with agents to reduce the stickiness of platelets in the blood. Aspirin and other antiplatelet agents are used. These agents seem to work best in the arterial circulation which is a high velocity and high-pressure setting.

Where blood pools in slow-flow areas, such as in the legs (during periods of immobility) and in the left atrial appendage (during periods of atrial fibrillation), the antiplatelet agents are far less effective and so anticoagulants are used for treatment. Heparin, low molecular weight heparin, warfarin and the Non-vitamin K Oral AntiCoagulants (NOACs, also an acronym for Novel Oral AntiCoagulant) reduce the risk of, or treat, clots that form in these slow-flow and low-pressure settings.

The 2017 COMPASS Study[9] asked the question: Can we have an each-way bet, putting patients on some aspirin and some anticoagulant, in particular the NOAC rivaroxaban? *In a group of high risk patients, the study demonstrated that having a bet each way was a successful approach, working particularly well within the group of people on which it was tested who had bad arteries in their legs.*

IMPORTANT POINTS   CLOTS

- Clots are needed to stop us from bleeding. **Good**.

- They can form when we don't want them to do so. **Bad**.

- They can develop in different locations in the body and are treated differently depending on where they form. **Tricky**.

---

[9]   COMPASS (Cardiovascular Outcomes for People Using Anticoagulation Strategies) New England Journal of Medicine 2017; 377:1319-1330

Atrial fibrillation is an increasing, worldwide problem with higher prevalence in the Western world. Let's see who is susceptible to developing this seemingly unpredictable condition.

Chapter 2 -
WHO SUFFERS FROM AF AND WHY?

Men suffer from atrial fibrillation as do women. Looking at the numbers[10], more men develop the disease; however, women, when they suffer the condition, run a higher risk of complications, including death. Although there is an increasing incidence of the condition as people age, young people, even as young as in their teens, can suffer from it, although this is uncommon.

In coming to a better understanding of atrial fibrillation, it is valuable to understand AF associations. To do this, we must distinguish that associations, the factors that lend weight to the possibilty of atrial fibrillation being present, are not causations, that is the mechanisms that give rise to the actual problem.

Let's look at this from outside the medical field. We know that speeding and alcohol consumption are significant associations with car accidents. However, we also know that people do drive over the speed limit with high alcohol levels yet do not have an accident. Conversely, we know that people who drive safely can be involved in an accident. This does not mean that driving within the speed limit and not consuming alcohol when driving is a waste of time. It simply alters the risk profile. It means that speed and alcohol are **associations** with having an accident. If they were causations, then every time someone sped or had consumed alcohol, that person would be involved in a car accident.

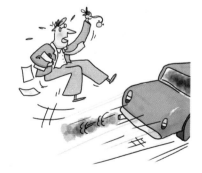

To take this a step further, alcohol does not cause the car accident; it does not drive the car, yet it can impair the driver's reflexes and assessment, and contribute to the driver having an accident. The actual cause of the accident may be approaching a sharp bend too quickly or a car in front stopping suddenly, while multiple associations may be present such as alcohol, speeding, driver inexperience, poor weather. The reverse may also be true. There may be no alcohol, no speeding or any other association, and still an accident occurs.

atrial fibrillation associations

Atrial fibrillation associations are found within the heart structure as well as externally.

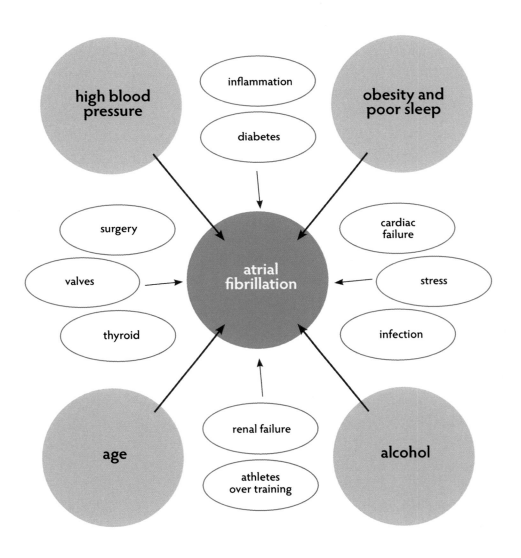

AF associations

within the heart

high blood pressure

the pressure changes caused by high blood pressure stretch the left atrium which, over time, will change the shape of the atrium, increasing the likelihood of it developing an abnormal rhythm. The change of shape is often also associated with

micro scarring

that changes the way the electricity flows through the atrium.

These factors along with

general wear and tear

increase the possibility of the electrical signal within the atria being deranged;

problems with the valves

also affect the pressures within the heart, again impacting the atrium's structure and subsequently its function, while

abnormality of the myocardium,

cardiac failure (including congenital heart problems)

can be similarly implicated.

outside the heart

obesity

particularly when it leads to

obstructive sleep apnoea

a condition in which the respiratory system is obstructed at night while the sufferer snores, producing low levels of oxygen within the bloodstream. This triggers a very brisk response from the sympathetic autonomic nervous[11] system that can increase blood pressure and can drive scarring and inflammation within the heart;

diabetes

long-term diabetes seems to impact the heart, possibly with by-products of diabetic metabolism ending up within the structure and the fibres of the myocardium, again affecting how the atria work;

chronic renal disease

nearly 20 percent of people with poor kidney function will develop atrial fibrillation, caused by elevated blood pressure, inflammation and a general propensity to scarring and change within the heart;

external toxins such as alcohol

regular consumption of too much alcohol has a strong association with the development of AF. A boozy night out, followed by bad sleep and a lot of snoring can trigger enough stimulation of the heart to kick off an episode of atrial fibrillation. Not uncommonly, people will present on Monday morning with a 'Saturday night arrhythmia' from just that!

thyroid problems

elevated abnormal levels of thyroid hormone can mimic the autonomic nervous system and contribute to development of atrial fibrillation;

infections and inflammation

pancreatitis is known to lead to atrial fibrillation, as is severe pneumonia or a severe infection of any sort, as the body responds to extra adrenaline created by the extra nervous activity occurring within it. It appears that anything within the body that increases the sympathetic autonomic nervous system can trigger an episode;

emotional stress

it is not uncommon to see patients who, for various reasons, have had a significant emotional incident which they have, literally, felt in their heart, with their heart jumping and fluttering. That emotional stressor has been the precipitant for atrial fibrillation to occur in that individual;

surgery

any surgery can act as a stressor on the heart; however, very commonly any surgery on the heart itself, in which the atria are actually handled during the process, markedly increases the risk of the development of AF;

pulmonary

importantly, after surgery or extended immobilisation, deep vein thrombosis can form in the legs. If these clots break off and flow back to the heart, they can pass through the right side of the heart and straight into the lungs. This is called a **P**ulmonary (pertaining to the lungs) thrombo**E**mbolism (a blood clot that moves through the bloodstream), PE, and can be life threatening. It can also be a trigger for atrial fibrillation. So, a post-operative patient who develops AF needs PE considered as a matter of priority;

genetic predisposition

there are certain families for whom a genetic link can have a significant up-regulation of the likelihood of someone within that family developing the condition, and interestingly,

endurance training

it is accepted that exercise in general is very good for a person's health and that normal levels of moderate exercise, several times a week, will lower the risk of heart-related illness and, in fact, lower the risk of atrial fibrillation.

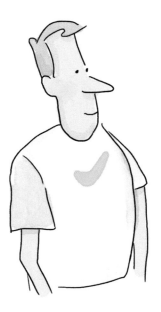

However, endurance athletes who undergo long, protracted training sessions for ultra events have been shown to run a higher risk of developing atrial fibrillation over time.

This is related to endurance activity leading to prolonged, increased cardiac output and subsequent increased size of the cardiac chambers as an adaptation. Neurologically, the heart responds with a tendency towards the parasympathetic nervous system[12] which seems to lower the threshold for the development of atrial fibrillation.

So, quite surprisingly, the last group of people impacted by atrial fibrillation are highly (perhaps, over) trained athletes.

what can be done about it?

Advancing age will lower a person's threshold to the development of atrial fibrillation, regardless of any other considerations. As age cannot be avoided, it is something that we can do little about. However, issues such as blood pressure, weight, good sleep, intake of alcohol and emotional stress are all controllable. Being aware of problems that can be associated with atrial fibrillation is a really important first step towards avoidance or management of the condition.

IMPORTANT POINTS ASSOCIATIONS

- The **big** three associations are obesity, high blood pressure and alcohol; all can be modified by the patient.

- The one we can't control is age.

- Associations all cause strain on the body and particularly the heart.

- AF can be a common final pathway of stress within the body.

---

[10] *2016 ESC Guidelines for the management of atrial fibrillation developed in collaboration with EACTS;* European Heart Journal *(2016) 37.2893-2962; page 2899*

In 2010, the estimated numbers of men and women with AF worldwide were 20.9 million and 12.6 million, respectively.

[11] *the 'flight or fight' nervous system at times of stress and emotion*

[12] *the 'rest and digest' system which conserves energy*

post-operative

Karen was a 75-year-old woman when I first met her. She was generally fit, well and active. She had had surgery for a colorectal problem. In the post-operative period, she developed AF. I was called and over the phone I recommended some digoxin to slow the heart rate down and also some metoprolol to slow down the heart rate with the potential of reverting the atrial fibrillation back into sinus rhythm.

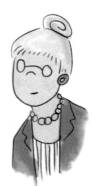

Before I saw her several hours later, clinically, she had returned to sinus rhythm. On speaking with her, it became clear that she had had episodes of palpitation in the past. I was comfortable in letting her go home on some regular metoprolol, hopefully to keep her out of trouble. I also put her on low-dose aspirin because she had just had surgery and I didn't want the risk of bleeding after the surgical procedure. I looked to review her in my rooms several weeks after her surgery and at that stage I also hoped to review her echocardiogram and Holter monitor testing.

The results of the echocardiogram showed that she had a dilated left atrium. This suggested that there was a reasonable chance she would have future recurrences of atrial fibrillation. That supported her reports of having had palpitations before the documented post-operative episode. The Holter monitor, which recorded the electrical activity of her heart over 24 hours, showed multiple episodes of short bursts of atrial ectopy, or extra beats arising from the atria. These can be a trigger for atrial fibrillation and for Karen they were occurring while she was on metoprolol. I was happy to keep her on metoprolol to try to dampen down the likelihood of the occurrence of palpitation.

She reported feeling really well and tolerated the metoprolol without issue. However, I thought there was a reasonable chance that, as time progressed, her AF threshold would reduce and, therefore, her likelihood of recurrence would increase. So, I swapped the aspirin to a NOAC to keep the blood thin. Karen was happy and she was well. We planned to touch base in six months to ensure that everything was travelling smoothly. So, Karen's post-operative atrial fibrillation was managed in the longer term on a beta-blocker (metoprolol) and anticoagulation, with regular follow-up planned.

Knowing about atrial fibrillation is one thing.
How is it diagnosed? Do you have it?

Chapter 3 -
DIAGNOSIS

Central to diagnosing atrial fibrillation is monitoring the electrical activity of the heart. So, before discussing the diagnosis of AF further, we need to understand in more detail the electrical activity as it passes through the heart and what 'normal' looks like. Then, we can look at the traditional, simplest and most convenient way of determining that the heart rhythm is normal or otherwise, and that is with an ECG.

*Remember, the **electrical activity** is what spreads through the heart muscle, leading to the **mechanical activity**, the pumping.*

the normal heart

As we have already seen, there are four main chambers within the heart: a right atrium (top)-ventricle (bottom) combination and a left atrium-ventricle combination. Blood flows from the body into the right side of the heart where it is pumped to the lungs for gas exchange before being returned to the left side of the heart to be pumped back around the body.

It is the right atrium (top right of the heart) in which the sinoatrial (SA) node acts as the heart's pacemaker, setting the beat for the rest of the heart.

All the cells of the heart have an automatic depolarisation system. This is called **automaticity**. This means that if you were to leave some of the cells out on a table, you could watch the cells contract as the electrical activity across the membrane changes. These cells leak sodium, potassium and calcium slowly and spontaneously until the charge across the membrane hits a threshold. When that threshold is reached, the change in the electrical potential over the membrane sets off an electrical trigger, called the action potential, which is the electrical depolarisation of the cell (lots of sodium and calcium flooding into the cell). This sets off the muscle fibrils and thereby, the contraction within those cells.

This is the 'electricity' of the heart. The cells in the sinoatrial node have the fastest tendency for this leakage so they have the fastest depolarisation cycle

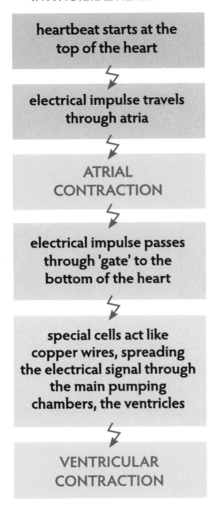

heartbeat starts at the top of the heart

electrical impulse travels through atria

ATRIAL CONTRACTION

electrical impulse passes through 'gate' to the bottom of the heart

special cells act like copper wires, spreading the electrical signal through the main pumping chambers, the ventricles

VENTRICULAR CONTRACTION

of any of the cells in the heart. That is why they set the beat.

Another really interesting thing about the muscle cells within the heart, over and above their having leaking membranes, is that they are all connected. Each cell connects to the next, to the next, to the next. This is achieved by special receptors between the cells that interlace and interconnect. This allows the electrical activity to flow rapidly through those cells. Those cells acting as one is called a **syncytium**.

When the sinoatrial node fires off, it leads to a wave of electrical activity (as we have said, not unlike a Mexican wave). Having started at the SA node, the wave moves from right to left through the atria.

Before flowing into the ventricles, the electrical activity has to pass through a fibrous ring that separates the atria and the ventricles. The fibrous ring does not allow the passage of electricity but has a special point where the electrical activity can travel from the top to the bottom of the heart. This is the **atrioventricular (AV) node**. This node acts as a gatekeeper and permits the electrical activity to pass from the atria to the ventricles, holding the passage for about one-tenth of a second. This ensures the ventricles beat after the atria.

Helping to distribute the electrical activity from the AV node through the ventricles are more specialised cells, Purkinje fibres, that act like copper wires. The heart contracts and then it goes back to normal. Remember the squid moving through the water: synchronous, coordinated, smooth. This is what the heart **should** do.

the ECG

An **ElectroCardioGram** (ECG) allows the electrical activity of the heart to be seen from different directions. Twelve electrodes monitor the electrical flow. The result is printed out or viewed on a screen.

The electrical activity in the atria is referred to as a **P wave** and it reflects atrial depolarisation or the electrical flow. As the electrical impulses pass through the AV node and then on to the special distribution cells, a **QRS complex** is created, reflecting the depolarisation of the major muscle of the heart. The last part of the electrical heartbeat is the **T wave** and this is the return of normal repolarisation to the heart muscle, ready for the next beat.

So, in the normal heart we see sinus rhythm, a beautiful synchronous atrial contraction followed by a beautiful synchronous ventricular contraction.

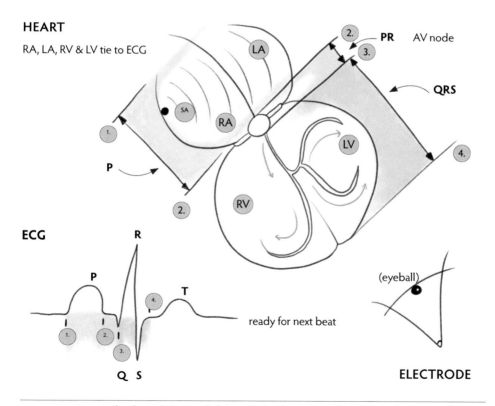

Imagine the electrode is an eyeball that sees the electrical impulse relative to the amount of current, with the current going to the electrode as an upright deflection or away, as a downward deflection. The P, Q, R, S and T waves show normal electrical flow.

In atrial fibrillation, the atria lose their synchronicity; the beats become chaotic and irregular. The AV node, the gateway to the electrical stimulation of the bottom of the heart, is bombarded by chaotic electrical activity, producing a heartbeat that is referred to as 'irregularly irregular'.

The atria are not working, the ventricles are beating in an irregular way and, so, the pump can't work properly.

When patients look at me blankly as I'm trying to explain 'irregularly irregular', I say that it is like someone who has no musical rhythm trying to dance; I think of myself perhaps a little intoxicated at those uni disco parties. Not cool!

P wave, sinus beat

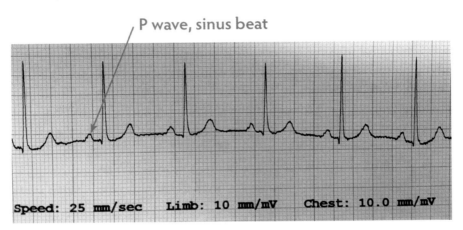

Speed: 25 mm/sec   Limb: 10 mm/mV   Chest: 10.0 mm/mV

no P wave

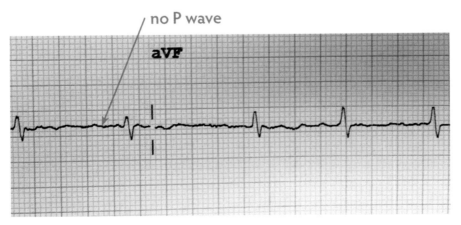

aVF

an ECG showing sinus rhythm (top) and atrial fibrillation (above)

diagnostic thumbprint

In a normal ECG, a P wave is followed by a QRS and a T. In atrial fibrillation there is no P wave. Instead, an ECG trace baseline shows bumps and irregularities and an occasional QRS complex from depolarisation reaching the ventricle, occurring irregularly and unpredictably.

This is our diagnostic thumbprint. Until we obtain a clear electrical tracing, we can't be sure of the rhythm.

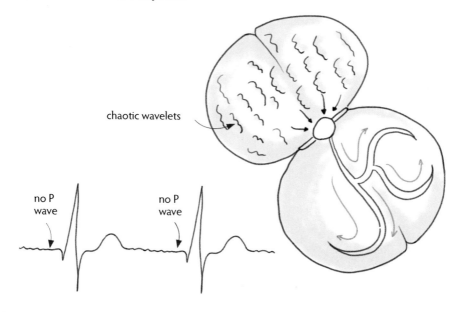

chaotic wavelets

no P wave

no P wave

irregular wriggly line of AF

beyond the ECG

The importance of obtaining an ECG trace to make the correct diagnosis explains why patients are asked to wear monitors for a time or have devices implanted for longer monitoring. It also helps to explain why the pulse sometimes needs to be checked in different ways.

Holter monitor

An ECG which monitors the heart for just a few minutes might not be long enough to establish if atrial fibrillation is present. If someone seems to be going in and out of atrial fibrillation with some regularity, maybe once or twice every couple of days, then the medical practitioner has the option to ask the patient to wear a monitor.

The monitor is a little box that the person can wear while undertaking normal daily activities such as being at home, at work, shopping, playing sport. It records electrical activity so that the medical practitioner can look for any irregularities that would establish an atrial fibrillation diagnosis. The result is not as detailed as from a 12-lead ECG, but it gives good information over a 24-hour, 48-hour or three-to-five-day period.

The most common monitoring, however, occurs in hospitals and is related to anaesthetic monitoring during surgery or monitoring undertaken in high dependency units. In these situations, finding atrial fibrillation is common and its appropriate care is important for the outcome for the patient.

implanted device

In some patients, there can be the suspicion that atrial fibrillation is occurring, but not frequently. If the cardiologist believes that the importance of making a diagnosis is high enough, then a very small device called a loop recorder *(pictured)* may be implanted under the skin above the heart.

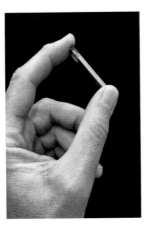

This really neat device can monitor the heartbeat 24-hours a day, seven days a week, for up to three years. The device is interrogated in a similar manner to a pacemaker, on a regular basis, using a special programmer that reads the data.

Patients can live a normal life while the device is implanted. The device does not go near a major organ; it is very simple to implant and take out and provides an incredible amount of data in relation to a suspected irregular rhythm that occurs very infrequently.

It is also worth remembering that pacemaker interrogation may also confirm the presence of atrial fibrillation.

pulse

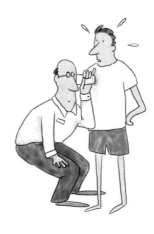

When a person's heartbeats are rapid and irregular and two or more beats come close together, the heart may not have had time to fill properly. Because the heartbeat is irregular, it means the filling of the ventricle, which takes time, will be variable; some beats will have more time to fill and some less. This results in more or less blood being pumped. Under these circumstances, the pulse won't necessarily be effectively felt at the wrist because the beats with 'less blood' may not be strong enough to be felt.

Similarly, it may be hard to measure the blood pressure as the beats will be of variable intensity.

Quite commonly, doctors who frequently deal with AF will measure the heartbeat by listening to the heart sounds at the apex of the heart which is on the left lateral border of the chest wall. However, the most accurate way is through an ECG. That way the medical practitioner can count exactly how many QRS complexes, or how many activations of the ventricle, are occurring in a given period.

IMPORTANT POINTS   DIAGNOSIS

- The cell membranes of the heart are leaky and as the SA node cells leak the fastest, they become the natural pacemaker.

- All the cells of the heart are connected and act as one; this is called a syncytium.

- The loss of the P wave, as shown on an electrical trace (ECG), confirms the diagnosis of atrial fibrillation.

- Loss of the P wave can be demonstrated
  - on a standard 12-lead ECG
  - through Holter monitoring in hospital or as an out-patient
  - by implanted devices used to monitor rhythm, and pacemakers.

ARE ALL PALPITATIONS ATRIAL FIBRILLATION?

The simple answer to this question is, "No; not every palpitation, not every irregular heartbeat, is atrial fibrillation".

Let's think of this in terms of palpitations or heartbeats that are either rapid and irregular, or rapid and regular.

rapid and irregular

When it comes to rapid and irregular heartbeats then atrial fibrillation, the chaotic electrical activity of the atrium giving rise to an erratic and irregular beat from the ventricle, is definitely the first possibility to consider. An irregular pulse, however, can be felt at the wrist as a consequence of other things.

P wave

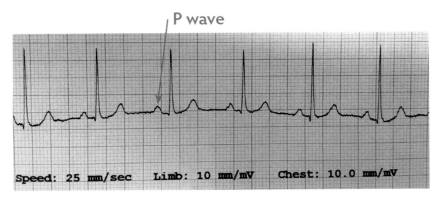

no P wave

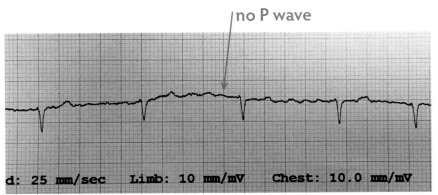

top: sinus rhythm   above: atrial fibrillation

We know that extra beats can arise in the top of the heart, from the atria, and also from the bottom of the heart, the ventricles. During normal beats, extra beats can slip in and give the illusion of irregularity. Extra beats arising from the top part of the heart are called **atrial ectopic beats**, atrial (top of the heart) ectopic (out of place) beat (heartbeat). So, atrial ectopic beats can give rise to irregularity of the pulse.

A similar process can occur in the ventricles. It is then called a **ventricular ectopic beat.**

Both atrial ectopic beats and ventricular ectopic beats can be felt by the patient because there is a change in rhythm. As the ectopic beat arises from a different location to where the atrium or the ventricle is normally activated, there is a discordant electrical impulse through the heart which results in a discordant contraction. Because of that, the heart moves in a different way from normal and the patient will often feel it.

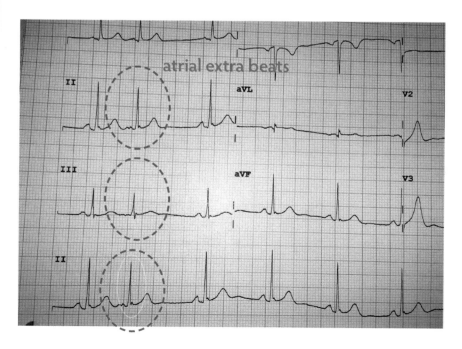

a heart in sinus rhythm yet showing atrial ectopic beats, or 'atrial extras'

So, an irregularity can arise from atrial ectopic beats or ventricular ectopic beats even though the patient may be in normal sinus rhythm.

rapid and regular

Rapid heartbeats can often be regular and this can point to a number of conditions.

It can be **atrial flutter** which is similar to atrial fibrillation except that there is a specific short circuit, called a re-entrant circuit, occurring in the right atrium. This sets a timing for the atrial rhythm at 300 bpm which is transferred to the ventricle at 150 bpm or fewer, due to the slowing down of the transmitted signals from the atria to the ventricles by the 'protective' AV node. If the AV node blocks every second impulse, we call this a 2:1 block.

The risks associated with atrial flutter are considered the same as for atrial fibrillation and both are treated similarly: rate control, anticoagulation and the possibility of restoration of normal sinus rhythm.

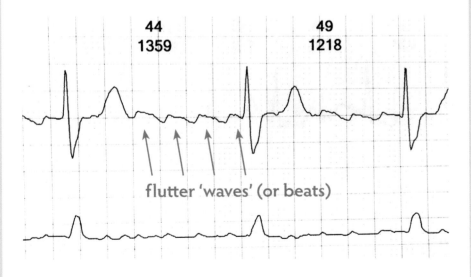

an ECG showing atrial flutter: the AV node in this example is
blocking 3 to 4 flutter beats for each impulse it lets pass to the ventricle, a 4:1 block

Another rapid regular rhythm is caused when a different type of re-entrant circuit forms within the atria. This re-entrant circuit, like atrial flutter, is an electrical short circuit, but in a different location. It also keeps going around and around, and firing on itself. This gives rise to a **supraventricular tachycardia**, supra (above the ventricle) tachy (fast) cardia (pertaining to heart).

Supraventricular tachycardia is a relatively common condition. It can give rise to heart rates of over 150 bpm and it often carries a different set of consequences to atrial fibrillation and atrial flutter.

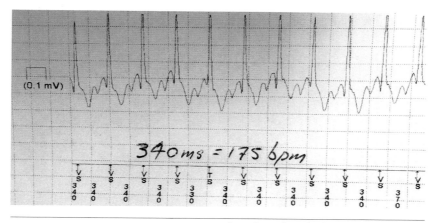

supraventricular tachycardia picked up on a loop recorder

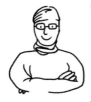

As we tend to see it in younger patients, doctors will often have a lower threshold to attempt a cure by using electrophysiological ablation rather than drug therapies for treatment.

Rapid rhythms that arise in the ventricle are very serious.

Ventricular tachycardia, *that the patient feels, is not common but it is a high-risk rhythm. Once the bottom part of the heart, the main pumping chamber of the heart, is beating rapidly in an abnormal rhythm, potentially we have problems.*

Ventricular fibrillation *is not felt. This is a rhythm that is not compatible with life. In atrial fibrillation, with the top part of the heart not working properly, the function of the pump is diminished but the ventricle still works. In ventricular fibrillation, when the main pumping chamber of the heart goes into chaotic rhythm, it just doesn't work at all. This is a cause of sudden cardiac death.*

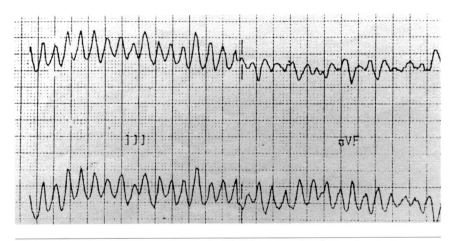

ventricular fibrillation is not compatable with life and is a cause of sudden cardiac death

What happens once an atrial fibrillation diagnosis is confirmed?

HOW

THE TREATMENT

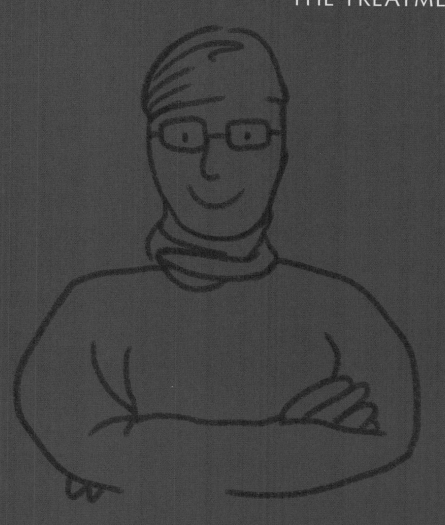

Chapter 4 -
INFORMATION

gathering information

Once atrial fibrillation is confirmed on the electrical trace, there is much more information to be gathered. What is going on within the patient's life and within the patient's heart that we can tie to atrial fibrillation?

It is easy to see if the patient is over-weight. We also want to assess the individual for diabetes, alcohol intake, sleep, blood pressure, thyroid function, stress and then we want to know about the structure of the heart, the function of the valves and the pressures within the heart and the lungs.

Importantly, we need to know the size of the atria. The bigger the atria, the greater the risk that the condition will recur. If the atria are normal size and the structure is normal, there is a good chance that the patient's heart can be returned to normal rhythm.

An **echocardiogram** (echo, sound; cardio, heart; gram, picture) or ultrasound of the heart will not only give a good appreciation of the **size of the atria**, but also the **size of the ventricles** and **how well they are working**. If there are conditions such as cardiac failure, features of longstanding hypertension or anything that could be wrong with the muscle, these are important factors to add to management strategy decisions for the individual.

The echo will also look at the **valves** in the heart. The aortic valve, the mitral valve, the pulmonary valve and the tricuspid valve are all important to our understanding of the patient's atrial fibrillation.

Particularly significant is the **mitral valve**, the valve between the left atrium and the left ventricle. If this valve is affected, for example narrowed or leaking excessively, then back pressure is directed immediately into the left atrium. This is significant when making management strategy decisions.

If the mitral valve is narrowed, thus slowing flow through the atrium, this is referred to as **'valvular' atrial fibrillation** and is associated with a greater risk of a clot forming in the left atrial appendage. It is also a factor in treatment selection, which will be discussed later.

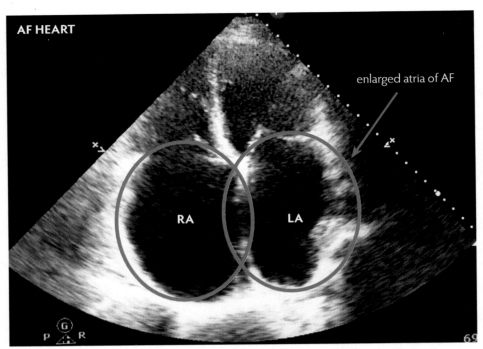

AF HEART

enlarged atria of AF

RA   LA

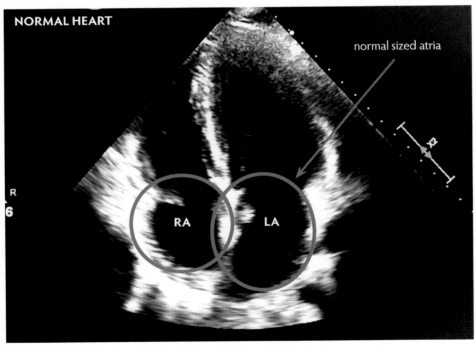

NORMAL HEART

normal sized atria

RA   LA

an echocardiogram, or ultrasound of the heart, shows heart structure and valves, and in the top photo, dilated atria due to long-standing atrial fibrillation

The ultrasound also looks at **pressures** within the heart. Are pressures elevated or are they normal? We look at pressures within the lungs too, also measured using ultrasound, as this gives an idea of the health of the remainder of the vascular system, including pulmonary vascular function.

In addition to confirming the diagnosis electrically and seeing the structure of, and function within, the heart, **blood tests** are also important at this stage. A thyroid function blood test is done routinely as it is known that increased thyroid hormone levels can be associated with initiating atrial fibrillation. Blood tests also allow us to determine if other problems are present. These could be sepsis, or inflammation, or illnesses such as anaemia which are known to be associations of atrial fibrillation.

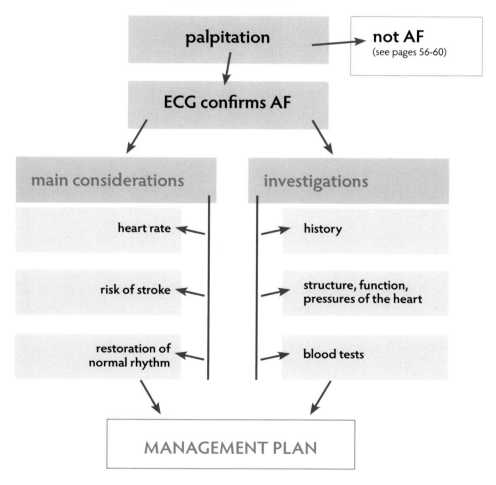

information needed to develop management strategies

considerations

Once atrial fibrillation has been diagnosed and the relevant associated information for the patient has been gathered, there are three areas of focus for AF management: heart rate, risk of stroke and if the patient should be returned to normal rhythm.

heart rate

Because of the chaotic beat within the atria, the heart is racing, often as fast as 150 and sometimes over 200 bpm, irregularly. This is very distressing to the person. At this rate, the heart doesn't work or fill properly so the speed needs to be slowed.

risk of stroke

Risk of stroke is of concern because, when the atria are not contracting properly, blood can pool, particularly in the left atrial appendage. Where it pools, a clot can form. Should this happen, the clot can find its way to the brain, leading to a catastrophic outcome, a stroke. To lower this risk, the blood needs to be 'thinned'. As part of the management strategy, especially around anticoagulant therapy, we utilise the CHA2DS2-VASc score, a clinical predictor for estimating the risk of stroke in patients with AF. Then, to determine the risk of complications from bleeding, another score, HAS-BLED, is used. *(For further information, please refer to pages 80 and 81.)*

returning the heart to sinus rhythm

A number of factors come into play in the decision of whether or not an attempt should be made to bring the person's heart back to normal, or sinus, rhythm.

understanding risk-benefit

Before elaborating on various treatments that are available, it is important to understand the concept of risk-and-benefit in relation to therapy. There is no medication available that has zero risk, so it is essential that patients be clear about what any risk might be. However, risk needs to be put into the context of the benefit, and benefit generally needs to be considered in the light of two different components: the **symptomatic** benefit (improving the way the patient feels) and the **prognostic** benefit (improving the long-term outcome).

In the case of **symptomatic** intervention for atrial fibrillation, if the patient's heart rate can be reduced, it will improve that patient's symptoms. So, the risk of the heart rate medication is weighed against the improved symptoms and better quality of life for the individual.

As the therapy is implemented, checks are done to ensure there really is a benefit. If we have improved the symptoms without unacceptable drug side-effects, then the benefit outweighs the risk for that individual and it's a reasonable intervention.

An example of a **prognostic** intervention for atrial fibrillation would be to give the person an anticoagulant to reduce the risk of stroke. This carries the risk of increased bleeding. It is also likely that thinning the blood doesn't make patients feel any better; they may even feel worse if they have problems with the medication.

So, ironically, patients may go for years thinking the prognostic medication has not done anything. Yet, the fact they have managed for so long probably means that the medication has worked very well and has been beneficial to them. "But I don't feel any different" is exactly the long-term goal for which we are aiming.

So, the risk-benefit has to be weighed against associated conditions such as cardiac failure, hypertension, increasing age, diabetes. Has the patient previously had a stroke? These factors point to the patient being at very high risk. Therefore he or she should derive a good deal of benefit from anticoagulation medication.

However, if the person is prone to tripping, has a history of self-harm with medications or is poor at taking medication, then the risk of using a blood thinning medication, perhaps, is unacceptable.

The bottom line is, is the risk of bleeding outweighed by the reduction in the risk of stroke for this person?

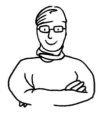

It is really important to understand that all medications will carry some risk; yet, there will also be benefits.

This risk-benefit discussion is an important one to have in any situation in which medication is being prescribed.

long-term tweaking

Francesca is a patient I have looked after for more than a decade. She was in her mid-to-late 60s when I first met her.

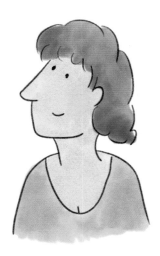

Francesca had had an episode of atrial fibrillation, somewhat unexpectedly. Her heart appeared structurally normal and she developed her symptoms without any clear-cut precipitant. In the early stages, she started aspirin and tried the beta-blocker, metoprolol. This didn't do the job and metroprolol was changed to sotalol which works through a slightly different mechanism. A follow-up at that time included investigation through the use of a Holter monitor. This showed that she was getting a number of extra beats within the atrium, beats called atrial ectopic beats or atrial ectopics. I find these atrial ectopics can sometimes respond well to calcium channel blockers and so I elected to swap Francesca to a relatively low dose of verapamil. It worked reasonably well. That was 2009.

After several months, she came back with a brief recurrence of palpitation. I added in a small dose of flecainide to her therapy regime. This seemed to do the job for Francesca and I didn't see her for more than two years. In that time her heart was structurally normal; she was not having atrial fibrillation; she had no other significant risk factors and was being appropriately managed with aspirin, verapamil and flecainide.

She came back in 2011. The recurrence of atrial fibrillation was no surprise as we expect AF to return, eventually. While we don't have a magic bullet to fix it, we do aim to control it.

In 2011 I gave her some instructions for a 'pill in a pocket' approach to deal with the recurrence of her AF and really, that worked pretty well over the next two to three years with only a couple of episodes occurring each year. During that time, she would take some extra flecainide, just to dampen down those episodes which were over within an hour or two. It would be fair to say that Francesca could worry herself into an episode of atrial fibrillation and more often than not, these episodes were associated with stressful events or situations in her life.

In 2013, she came back again. The latest episodes had been short-lived, occurring very infrequently with no more than one episode every few months. I increased the verapamil dosage slightly and we waited to see how things would progress. In the course of the next year, we increased the dosage of both the verapamil and the flecainide, just a little.

The way I describe that, the up-titration or increasing the dose, is a little bit like adding salt to a casserole. You don't want to pour a whole tub of salt in because you can spoil the dish. You really want to add in just what's required, no more, no less. And so, bringing patients back and adding in just a little allows us to creep up the dose so that we are meeting the needs of the patient by reducing the recurrence of the arrhythmia, but we are not giving the patient more than is needed.

In 2017, which was the next time Francesca came back, she was having only intermittent, short-lived episodes. However, she was by then nearly 10 years older and I was concerned about the recurrence of atrial fibrillation in someone who would have been at increased risk from atrial fibrillation-induced stroke.

We had the conversation about anticoagulation. Francesca started on one of the new NOAC agents available, rivaroxaban.

While she still has short-lived episodes infrequently, she is really comfortable on her current therapy using verapamil and flecainide and she is tolerating the NOAC without any problems. A Holter monitor follow-up showed she was having less than 0.5 percent of her day in atrial fibrillation. So, the anticoagulant was making her safe and the antiarrhythmics were keeping her symptom-free for the vast majority of the time.

In very recent times she has described a little shortness of breath. A follow-up echocardiogram showed that her pulmonary pressures had snuck up a little bit. This meant her body may have been retaining a little bit too much fluid in the circulation. This was not surprising. As people get older their heart can become stiffer. This stiff heart sends messages to the kidneys that something is 'just not right' and this tends to lead to fluid retention. This fluid can build up in the lungs and manifest as shortness of breath. So, we introduced some diuretic *therapy[13] just to take the fluid off on an as-needed basis. Voila, symptomatic success!*

Francesca is now travelling really well. It has been 10 years of atrial fibrillation for her and over that time there have been some changed medications; we've up-titrated medications; we've given her a 'pill in the pocket'; we've moved from aspirin as a preventative for risk of stroke to an anticoagulant and we are monitoring the flecainide with regular ECGs.

Francesca, who has been a great patient to work with over these years, is happy. She is appropriately covered from a prognostic perspective; she is symptomatically well, and her atrial fibrillation is well-controlled with the risks reduced by the anticoagulant.

IMPORTANT POINTS   INFORMATION

Following ECG confirmation of atrial fibrillation

- **gather information**
  - history
  - echo
  - bloods

- **treatment**
  - slow the heart rate
  - reduce the risk of stroke
  - consider restoration of sinus rhythm
  - understand the risk-benefit of any medication

---

[13]   *A diuretic makes the person pass urine.*

Now it is time to look at the 'how' of the various treatments available.

Chapter 5 -
How do we SLOW THE HEARTBEAT?

When a patient is seen in an acute setting, for example, having presented at an accident and emergency department, or is being seen by the cardiologist for the first time, often his or her heart rhythm is rapid and quite distressing for the person. By slowing down the heart rate, it makes the patient feel better and improves the working of the heart, so it is a good starting point and one to be addressed as soon as possible.

beta-blockers

There are a number of drugs used to control the heart rate. The most commonly used drugs are from a group called beta-blockers. They act through receptors that are associated with the sympathetic nervous system. These receptors are normally used to accelerate the nervous system within the body, giving us the 'fight and flight' response which increases the heart rate, dilates the pupils (for seeing better), increases blood flow to the muscles (to run away or fight) and increases blood pressure.

Beta-blockers act to impede these receptors. In effect, **the beta-blockers dampen the sympathetic nervous system which has nerve endings supplying the atrioventricular (AV) node,** thus reducing the speed of AF conduction from the atria to the ventricles and so slowing the heart rate.

However, beta-blockers can also lower blood pressure. This needs to be monitored closely. If the patient already has low blood pressure, it may mean that beta-blockers cannot be used. Beta-blockers can occasionally stir up asthma and some patients will describe fatigue and, infrequently, depression. Occasionally, though, I've had patients tell me they feel great, being more centred and grounded.

For most people, these agents are flexible and work well and are often used as the first-line agent in treating atrial fibrillation. They can be administered either orally, in tablet form, or intravenously, through the vein. One commonly used agent is **metoprolol.**

digoxin

Depending on the heart rate response to the first line of therapy, beta-blockers can be used in conjunction with other medications or other medications are used instead of the beta-blockers. One of the agents I like to use, often in conjunction with beta-blockers, is **digoxin**.

Digoxin, which is derived from digitalis which comes from the foxglove plant, acts to **slow the atrioventricular node**, thus slowing the ventricular rate. This leads to improved control.

On the positive side, digoxin is often very well-tolerated and does not tend to lower blood pressure. On the negative side, there can be problems if the patient's kidneys are not working well as the drug can accumulate in the body if used longer-term. Its use must be monitored closely.

Digoxin can be administered orally or intravenously. Used alone or in combination with beta-blockers, it can work very effectively to bring down the heart rate.

calcium channel blockers

If choosing not to use beta-blockers, say for a patient with asthma, another option is a centrally acting calcium channel blocker. A calcium channel blocker is an agent that affects the way calcium flows through the cell membrane; a centrally-acting calcium channel blocker is one that acts predominantly on the heart compared with a peripherally-acting agent that has more effect on the blood vessels.

Verapamil and **diltiazem** are centrally-acting agents.

Although verapamil is probably used more often, both **regulate ventricular reaction**, slowing the response in atrial fibrillation, again through slowing the gateway between the atria and the ventricles, the AV node.

Care needs to be taken in their use by people who already have problems with their left ventricular function.

Each can be given as a tablet or through the vein.

amiodarone

While beta-blockers, digoxin and calcium channel blockers are the main agents for rate control, in certain **emergency circumstances**, amiodarone might be used.

Amiodarone is a separate sort of agent with a different class of antiarrhythmic effect. It can be given orally; however, because it takes a long time to build up its levels within the body, it is far more effective in the acute setting if given intravenously. This agent, on its own, can slow down the atrial fibrillation rate. It is also a powerful reversion (returning the patient to normal rhythm) agent. So, its use can start to slow the heart with the possibility of returning the patient to normal rhythm.

On the downside, it carries a lot of iodine that can affect the thyroid gland in the long-term. In up to 25 percent of patients thyroid problems will develop. Amiodarone can also lead to toxicity within the lungs and the liver, and cause skin pigmentation.

While it is not at the top of the list for controlling heart rate, it should not be overlooked. If needed, it should be used with care.

BETA-BLOCKER	dampens sympathetic nervous system	metoprolol (common agent)
	care: can lower blood pressure, can cause asthma *administer:* orally or intravenously	
DIGOXIN	slows the AV node so slows ventricular rate	
	care: monitor levels *administer:* orally or intravenously	in conjunction with beta-blockers or on its own
CALCIUM CHANNEL BLOCKERS	regulate ventricular reaction by slowing the AV node	verapamil (more common) diltiazem
	care: existing problems with left ventricular function *administer:* orally or intravenously	
AMIODARONE	emergency circumstances	
	care: iodine levels, thyroid, toxicity *administer:* orally, although intravenous better in acute settings	can lead to cardioreversion

TACHYCARDIA-INDUCED CARDIOMYOPATHY

Tachy means fast; cardia and cardio relate to the heart and myopathy refers to a problem with the muscle. So, tachycardia induced cardiomyopathy is a fast heart induced muscle problem.

This can tie in with atrial fibrillation. We see it most commonly in people who have silent, persistent atrial fibrillation; the patient is not necessarily aware of the rhythm and it lasts for an extended time, of weeks to months.

*The normal heart rate is between 50 and 100 bpm. If the heart is being driven rapidly over its normal rate, say in the 130s, 140s, 150s or even above that, the heart suffers. Over time, it shows features of fatigue: dilating and not contracting as effectively as it should do. This is **cardiomyopathy;** the muscle of the heart becomes fatigued and 'wears out'. If this is not treated, it can lead to heart failure and death.*

By the time we see these people, the development has been gradual. They are often short of breath and their heart rate is very fast. They have a dilated heart which we can pick up on clinical examination and on ECG and even more clearly on echocardiography. They have features of heart failure and respond well to the standard therapies that have an emphasis on rate control.

Different factors may have caused the heart to dilate. Infection may have damaged the heart muscle, giving rise to an infective cardiomyopathy. The person may have consumed too much alcohol, an alcoholic cardiomyopathy. It may be related purely to the heart rate being too fast. Sometimes, we can't be sure of the cause. Nonetheless, one of our therapy mainstays is to slow down the heart rate.

If we reduce that heart rate effectively, starting to bring it back towards the 70-odd beats per minute which is normal, then often we can see a fantastic response. Some patients respond even better if we are able to restore sinus rhythm. (Please see chapters 7 and 8.)

The really satisfying thing about this condition is that if we can slow down the heart rate of these people for several months, say three months, they will come back feeling much better and a re-evaluation of their hearts shows marked improvement in function. It is a very satisfying outcome.

IMPORTANT POINTS SLOWING THE HEART RATE

- We slow the heart rate by slowing the electrical activity passing through the AV node, the node that allows electrical impulses to pass from the atria to the ventricles.

- Drug therapies to do this are
  - beta-blockers
  - digoxin
  - calcium channel blockers
  - amiodarone.

How do we thin the blood?

Chapter 6 -
How do we THIN THE BLOOD?

Strategies for thinning the blood are important in the treatment and management of atrial fibrillation as risk of stroke is a serious consideration. The pooling of blood in an atrium that is not contracting properly can lead to the formation of a clot within the left atrium, specifically in a recess called the left atrial appendage. Should this clot be dislodged, it can pass through the left ventricle, make its way to the brain and cause a stroke. Thinning the blood reduces that risk.

Before considering situations in which it is important to thin the blood, let's look at how a blood clot forms and understand the coagulation cascade, both important factors in understanding atrial fibrillation treatment.

protection

The body needs to be able to protect itself if there is damage to the circulation. If bleeding from a cut or a scratch is not stopped, the person will bleed to death. The mechanism that stops us bleeding to death is the formation of a blood clot, or thrombosis.

The coagulation cascade, in its simplest terms, has two major components that give rise to the formation of a clot. One component is the small particles that come from the bone marrow and are called **platelets.** They don't have a nucleus, so they are not 'complete' cells but they are part of what forms a clot. The other element, in conjunction with platelets, is a strong cross-bridging strand protein called **fibrin,** the scaffold of the clot formation.

When there is damage to the blood vessel, proteins and receptors that are not normally exposed to the blood circulation become exposed. With this, platelets come into contact with receptors with which they normally would not have contact. Those proteins and receptors activate platelets, causing changes which lead to preparation for forming a clot. So that fibrin is formed to bind with those platelets, a cascade of different factors is started. That cascade is called the **coagulation cascade.** The clot formation occurs through the activation of platelets which results in the platelets interacting with fibrin, after the fibrin has been generated through the coagulation cascade. In atrial fibrillation, the main driver is stasis of blood, or stagnation of the normal flow of blood, within the left atrial appendage, allowing clotting factors to interact in a way that is just not possible when they are in free-flowing blood within the circulation.

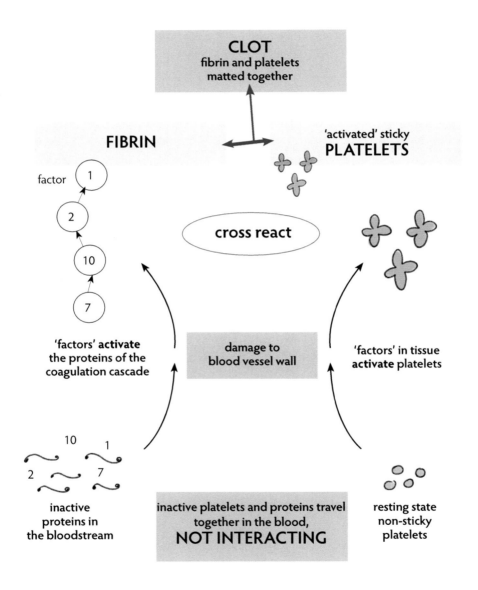

simplified schematic of the formation of a blood clot

Fibrin and platelets together form the clot that blocks or seals the blood vessel.

What then stops the clot progressing until all the blood congeals?

So that the whole body doesn't end up as one big clot, there are also factors generated that limit the progression of a clot. These factors are called the **fibrinolytic system**. As the body is forming a clot, it is also producing factors that prevent the clot from extending too far.

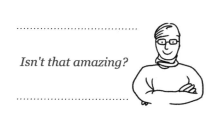

Isn't that amazing?

In some medical situations, such as atrial fibrillation and other heart-related matters, the body does not want a clot to form as it can cause a more serious problem, such as a stroke or a heart attack. To help stop a clot forming, **anti-coagulation therapies** are implemented, keeping in mind two major risks: the possibility of stroke in the future and the likelihood of bleeding.

It is important to understand something about the clot-forming pathway as it helps patients understand where and why medications work. For example, aspirin and clopidogrel are used to dampen down platelet function. Warfarin, heparin and the NOACs are used to work on the coagulation cascade. These different agents act in different locations within the clotting cascade, essentially to decrease the production of the end product, the fibrin, and so reduce the possibility of a clot forming.

fibrin

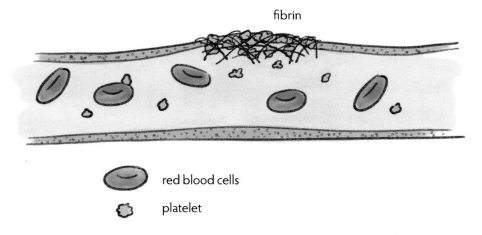

red blood cells

platelet

structure of a blood clot

KEEPING SCORE: CHA$_2$DS$_2$-VASc and HAS-BLED

There are two significant considerations that come into play when deciding on anticoagulation therapy:

- *risk of stroke in the future*

- *risk of bleeding.*

A risk score calculator has been developed for each of these considerations.

risk of having a stroke	risk of bleeding on anticoagulation
CHAD SCORE	HAS-BLED SCORE

balancing risks

*People who suffer **C**ardiac failure, high blood pressure (**H**ypertension), increasing **A**ge and **D**iabetes (CHAD) all have an increased risk of stroke if they also have atrial fibrillation. A tool has been formulated in which these parameters receive a score. The tally of those scores is then used in management decisions. Over time, the original CHAD score has been modified with more information being added.*

Today's CHA2DS2-VASc score offers extra options: age variability (it breaks down age groups into lower, intermediate and higher risks), the patient's sex (women run a higher risk of stroke), and it also adds, as a consideration, previous stroke or vascular disease within the arterial system. As these parameters provide a likelihood of the risk of stroke in the future, the score is used in decision-making regarding the need for anticoagulation therapy.

Should the patient need anticoagulation therapy, the question then needs to be asked, How safe is anticoagulant therapy for that patient? with the consideration here being the risk of bleeding.

Here, we look at another score, HAS-BLED: **H**ypertension, **A**bnormal renal or liver function, previous **S**troke, previous **B**leeding problems principally from the gut, **L**abile control of warfarin (labile INR), **E**lderly (over 65 years of age), **D**rugs or alcohol. As with the CHA2DS2-VASc score, each parameter is given a score, with the tally indicating the risk of bleeding for that individual.

The HAS-BLED score was developed before the NOAC agents became widely available and so the labile INR can be removed from the score if a NOAC is to be used. However, if that is done, the medical practitioner needs to consider renal function as this is known to be a driver for risk of bleeding. Adequate renal function is needed for metabolism of the NOACs.

The CHA2DS2-VASc score and the HAS-BLED score are married to help to make a management decision for our patient based on the balance of where we think those scores lie. We try to weigh up the risks for the person the best we can. You will remember Gran from the introduction. In her case, the HAS-BLED score, or the risk of bleeding, was so high from the difficulties with warfarin that it outweighed the CHAD score, or the risk of having a stroke, and this was reflected in her treatment.

The risks need to be reviewed periodically as both scores can change with time. For example, the age component will increase, the cardiac failure component could change, high blood pressure could be brought under control or develop. Although these scores are dynamic, they give us a good understanding for trying to mitigate future risk of stroke and future risk of bleeding for the patient.

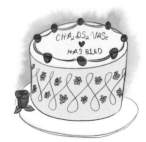

now and later

There are two different situations in which thinning the blood to reduce the risk of stroke can be considered: the acute setting when somebody first presents, and in the longer term.

In the **acute setting**, historically, drugs such as **heparin** and **clexane** which act on factor 10 in the clotting cascade, have been used. Both these drugs work effectively and can be given as injections as soon as a person presents at an accident and emergency department. The treating doctors will address atrial fibrillation by slowing the person's heart rate and dealing with the risk of stroke, simultaneously.

Heparin and clexane work well in this acute situation. However, because they are administered as injections either into the skin or into the vein, they are generally not practical, **long-term** solutions. Who would want ongoing injections as a treatment if there is a pill that can be swallowed?

warfarin

Warfarin is the blood thinner with which people are most familiar, at least by name. Some of my patients often refer to warfarin as 'rat killer' as it is the active ingredient in the substance used as rat poison for many, many years.

Historically, warfarin has been the go-to therapy.

In our bodies, warfarin blocks the action of vitamin K which is used by the liver to produce the clotting factors. Warfarin is not a good agent in the acute setting as it can take several days for the proteins that it blocks to be cleared from the system and therefore have its full effect. It also needs adjustment from patient to patient and over time.

new agents, NOACs

Another option is the use of new agents on the market, **D**irect or **N**ovel **O**ral **A**nti**C**oagulants, often referred to as DOACs or NOACs. These agents act directly on the coagulation cascade and each acts quickly. Most conveniently, these medications do not need regular blood tests to monitor their effect. However, in Australia specific criteria need to be met for them to be prescribed and funded by the Commonwealth Government[14]. NOACs include the drugs **apixaban**, **dabigatran** and **rivaroxaban**.

With the advent of these new agents, my practice now is to use them as soon as possible, including on a person's arrival at the accident and emergency department, unless there is any clear contraindication of their use. Within hours we see a result; blood thinning occurs. They can be used long-term and the NOACs do not require regular monitoring as does warfarin.

The limitation with these NOACs is that the patient needs to have good, or at least reasonable, renal function so that the drugs don't build up in the body and cause toxicity problems. In the situation in which the patient has significantly reduced renal function and will require long-term anticoagulation, then warfarin is the tried and tested option. While it does need to be monitored and adjusted on a regular basis, it works.

The NOACs are also specifically recommended for patients who have no significant heart valve problems. If a patient has a narrowing of the mitral valve, slowing flow between the atrium and the ventricle, or has had a mechanical heart valve replacement of any sort, even in the setting of good renal function, warfarin is the appropriate agent. An abnormality of the valves of this type is referred to as valvular AF, and NOACs are not recommended for this group of patients.

The NOAC agents have similarities and differences.

Apixaban and rivaroxaban both work through factor 10 which is the same factor through which heparin and clexane work. There is a sense within the medical fraternity that apixaban is slightly gentler for the older age group, particularly for people with slight renal impairment. Practical application suggests that the convenience of rivaroxaban as a single daily dose is preferred by patients.

Dabigatran works through factor 2. The outcomes are very similar to using apixaban and rivaroxaban. Dabigatran has a reversal agent, which can be an important factor in decision-making around the selection of the direct oral anticoagulant the doctor might choose for a person's atrial fibrillation.

Apixaban and rivaroxaban both have a reversal agent under development and it is likely to be available soon. A reversal agent is significant should the anticoagulation need to be stopped quickly, especially in an emergency situation.

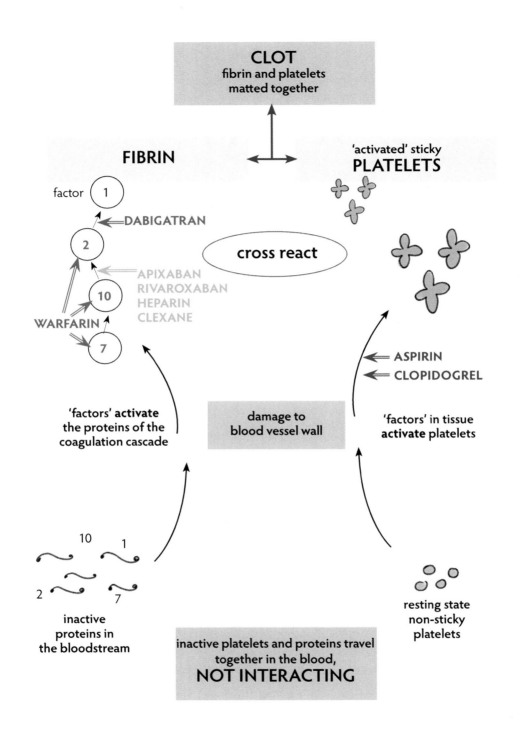

where blood thinning agents act in relation to the formation of a clot

WARFARIN

The adjustment of warfarin is a 'Goldilocks' process. We don't want the blood **too thin** (from too much warfarin), nor do we want the blood **too thick** (not enough warfarin). We want it **just right.**

We arrive at 'just right' by measuring the time it takes for the blood to form a clot in a special laboratory test. This test has been standardised worldwide and is called the **I**nternational **N**ormalised **R**atio (INR). This means you can have your INR checked anywhere in the world and know how to deal with the result.

When thinning blood for atrial fibrillation, we generally aim for an **INR of over two and less than three**. Too low will not be effective and too high will run an unacceptably high risk of bleeding.

Having an **INR under two or over three** is called being **out of therapeutic range**, that is, not in the range required for effective and safe therapeutic effect.

The way we achieve therapeutic warfarin levels, when someone is starting to use the drug, is generally to load the patient with highish doses for a couple of days, to start the blood thinning effect, and then check the effect using a blood test. The process then becomes one of increasing or lowering the dose to achieve the desired INR. This is called 'titrating' the dose and it can often take a few weeks before the correct level is achieved.

The objective is to find the ideal dose for the patient and then check the INR on a regular basis, perhaps monthly for a stable patient. Anyone on warfarin will need to become familiar with regular blood tests for checking their INR.

Recently, hand-held home devices have become available, allowing patients to adjust their own warfarin dose based on this home testing. This is a great solution for some people.

It is also really important to remember that the effect of warfarin may change based on external factors. Illness or, perhaps even more importantly, the addition of other drugs, can interact with warfarin and alter the INR, as can some foods. Change in a patient's clinical situation requires close attention to the INR to avoid complications.

	WARFARIN	NOAC
cost per tablet	CHEAP	EXPENSIVE
regular blood tests to adjust	YES	NO
altered by foods, particularly greens	YES	NO
interaction with other medications	YES, MANY	MINIMAL, FEW
severe renal failure	YES	NO
mild or moderate renal impairment	YES	YES
mechanical heart valves	YES	NO
mitral stenosis	YES	NO
time to onset	DAYS, NEEDS ADJUSTMENT	HOURS
reversal agent	NOT REALLY. VIT K IS TOO SLOW TO WORK TO BE EFFECTIVE	YES, FOR DABIGATRAN. LIKELY SOON FOR RIVAROXABAN & APIXABAN
effectiveness at blood thinning	OUT OF THERAPEUTIC RANGE UP TO 30 PERCENT OF THE TIME	BETTER
risk of bleeding	SIMILAR	SIMILAR, THOUGH LESS BLEEDING INTO BRAIN
tolerability, side-effects, discontinuation	SIMILAR	SIMILAR
overall costs	NEEDS TO INCLUDE THE DRUG, MONITORING, TIME THERAPY OUT OF RANGE, RATES OF BLEEDING AND RATES OF STROKE	PROVEN A COST-EFFECTIVE ALTERNATIVE WITH MORE CONVENIENCE, FEWER BLEEDING ISSUES, FEWER STROKES
use with stenting	YES	YES
impact on VIT K	YES	NO

WHAT IF I CAN'T TOLERATE WARFARIN OR NOACS?

A situation can arise when a patient may have clear reasons for not taking blood-thinning medications but still needs protection from the risk of stroke associated with AF. For example, a patient who may have an abnormality of blood vessels in the brain which could be at risk of bleeding, cannot be on a blood thinner.

There is a possible solution. The recent development of a rather audacious idea that, if you can block off the left atrial appendage (the recess in the left atrium), preventing the stagnant pooling of blood there, then perhaps you can prevent the formation of a clot altogether.

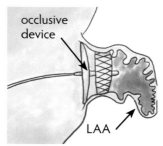

Several randomised studies have compared warfarin therapy with the use of an implanted left atrial occlusive device and found that the device worked just as well as warfarin. This means that, for really high-risk patients who just aren't able to take blood-thinning medications, there may be an alternative.

HOW DO I COPE WITH RECURRENT BLEEDING?

*Bleeding from the nose, called epistaxis, and bleeding from the bottom, called **P**er **R**ectal or PR bleeding, can be a real nuisance for some patients and each problem needs a solution.*

I try to deal with the underlying problem: cautery to the lining of the nose and ligation of haemorrhoids for bleeding piles. If these don't work then, perhaps, an alternate agent can be used, for example, warfarin to a NOAC, or a change of dose of the NOAC. This could be dabigatran 150 mg to 110 mg twice daily, rivaroxaban 20 mg to the 15 mg preparation, or maybe apixaban 5 mg to the 2.5 mg preparation.

The solution is a matter of finding a way that weighs risk against benefit and convenience against inconvenience.

SILVER LININGS TO ANTICOAGULATION RISKS

Although the advantage of thinning the blood is clear, it does carry risks.

When we thin the blood, we increase the risk of bleeding, particularly bleeding into the brain and also into the gut. So, the risk of a haemorrhagic stroke increases with the use of blood thinners and any lesions within the gut have a greater propensity to bleed.

Is there a silver lining to these increased risks? Are there other situations where the effect of blood thinners could be beneficial?

The one that comes immediately to mind is long distance travel and the potential to develop a clot in the leg. **Bad.** *This can lead to a pulmonary embolism if the clot moves to the lungs.* **Really bad.** *The possibility of this very serious condition developing can be mitigated by taking an anticoagulant.*

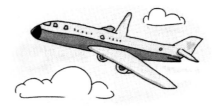

Is there a similar silver lining from increased risk of bleeding?

Over the years, I have seen a number of my patients who have had bowel cancer detected early because they were taking anticoagulants. This is how their increased propensity to bleed was a benefit.

One of the screening tests routinely used looks for evidence of blood in the bowl motion or stool. That blood is in the bowel motion because a problem in the bowel, the beginnings of a cancer, is scraped by the faeces moving past, causing bleeding and a small amount of blood ends up in the stool. This screening test is called a faecal (faeces) occult (not easily seen) blood test. If a person is on a blood thinner when one of the early cancers is rubbed, it is more likely to bleed, with the possible result of showing an abnormality.

Whether or not you are on warfarin or a NOAC, it might be a good time to ask your local doctor if you are due for a faecal occult blood test looking for an abnormality in the gut.

....

Catch bowel cancers as early as possible for the best chance of a good outcome.

It's also an interesting thought that maybe in the future, to try to increase the sensitivity of the test, that faecal occult blood testing could be combined with the person taking an anticoagulant, for a few days, before the test. I have not seen any data about this. However, it is an entertaining and potentially useful consideration.

....

IMPORTANT POINTS   THINKING THE BLOOD

- The coagulation cascade results in a 'plug' of platelets and fibrin.
- We thin the blood
    - **acutely**, with heparin, clexane, NOACs
    - **long-term**, with warfarin or NOACs.
- When using NOACs, there needs to be checks on kidney function and consideration of the valves of the heart.
- When using warfarin, there needs to be monitoring of the INR and consideration of possible interactions with other drugs, foods.
- Advent of the NOAC agents has reduced reliance on the use of warfarin.

---

[14]   *For NOACs to be prescribed and Government-funded in Australia, the patient must have non-valvular atrial fibrillation and one or more risk factors for developing stroke or systemic embolism. These include prior stroke, being 75 years or older, having hypertension, diabetes mellitus, heart failure and/or left ventricle ejection fraction 35 percent or less. (Pharmaceutical Benefits Scheme)*

One of my soapboxes is encouraging patients, especially those on blood thinners, to know the medications they are taking and to carry a list in case of an emergency.

Why?

Well, imagine if you are out, fall and end up unconscious. Do you think it would be helpful for your treating doctors at the hospital to find a list in your wallet that lets them know you are on an anticoagulant? Do you think it could save your life? You bet it could!

*So, **please, please, please,** always have an up to date list of medications in your wallet or purse. It will ensure you have the chance of receiving the best health care, especially in the case of an emergency.*

How do we bring the heart back to normal rhythm?

Chapter 7 -
How do we BRING THE HEART
BACK TO NORMAL RHYTHM?

Is bringing a patient's heart back to normal rhythm a treatment priority?

A patient's symptoms and that patient's risk of a stroke must be remembered when considering an attempt to keep the patient's heart in normal rhythm. To date, the vast majority of the research done into returning people to normal rhythm does **not** demonstrate an outcome benefit. It demonstrates a symptomatic benefit, in that people feel better within themselves in normal rhythm; yet, returning people to normal rhythm surprisingly does not reduce risk of an adverse event in the long-term.

That means that these people are still having strokes. Even if a person has been returned to normal rhythm, there is a very good chance that the person will continue to flip in and out of atrial fibrillation and so still be at risk of a clot forming in the left atrial appendage and therefore still be at risk of stroke. Controlling the rhythm alone is not enough, as it is just not 100 percent effective.

In many situations, even if there appears to be good rhythm control, it might be necessary to look at rhythm control in combination with anticoagulation so that the patient's symptoms and risk of stroke are covered together. Driven by the symptoms they are experiencing, many patients are quite attached to the idea of getting out of atrial fibrillation, sometimes by a feeling that 'it's just not right' or they simply want it 'fixed'.

My experience is that in a large number of patients for whom returning the heart to normal rhythm proves a difficulty, over time (probably six to 12 months) they gradually develop a tolerance to the presence of atrial fibrillation within their body. If we have controlled the rate so that the heart doesn't race too much, the patient eventually becomes used to the heart functioning in that altered way. The symptomatic control, which was quite a major consideration early in the management, becomes less significant over time. It is also important to remember that medications used to maintain sinus rhythm potentially also have side-effects. We don't want to push those too hard because the side-effects may become more trouble than the condition. As always, it comes down to an assessment of the pros and cons of any therapeutic strategy in relation to the individual patient.

timing

When looking to return a person to normal rhythm, importantly we try to ascertain **when** the person went into atrial fibrillation.

If a person presents **within 48 hours** of the onset of atrial fibrillation, the person can be returned to normal rhythm quickly, as long as there is no structural abnormality of the heart or any other coexisting conditions that could lead to any uncertainty around the safety of so doing. If we see a person within 48 hours, we will put that person on some anticoagulant to reduce the risk of the formation of a clot in the heart.

If the patient is seen **beyond 48 hours,** that person would be put on anticoagulation treatment for three to four weeks before making any attempt to restore normal rhythm. This is to ensure we minimise the risk of a clot being in the heart. The theory says that if we use anticoagulation, the fibrinolytic system (the clot break-down system) has a chance to clear that clot from the system. Remember, if we return normal contraction to the atria and there is a clot in the left atrial appendage, then the contraction may actually dislodge the clot.

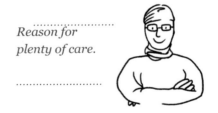

Reason for plenty of care.

Should it be decided to attempt to return a patient to sinus rhythm, there are two methods: **pharmacological**, using medications, and **electrical**, using electricity to restart the heart. Both can be used in the acute setting.

within 48 hours, pharmacological

Commonly, people present to accident and emergency for assessment with their first episode of atrial fibrillation. For the patient, there is quite a deal of apprehension associated with it. Medications used in this setting can be given either by mouth or through the vein. The most common agents used are beta-blockers, including metoprolol. Many cardiologists use flecainide, orally or through the vein, when patients have low blood pressure and it is unclear if they would tolerate beta blockade, they may be given amiodarone.

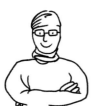

For patients who have previously been assessed and have structurally normal hearts, are not complicated medically and are symptomatic of their AF, then a 'pill in the pocket' regime can be employed, especially if they are having very infrequent episodes of atrial fibrillation. They implement the regime as soon as they are aware of the onset of atrial fibrillation.

That regime may include some beta-blockers, heart rate regulators or specific antiarrhythmics. Those patients may also have an anticoagulant tablet to take immediately, to ensure that the blood is thin should the 'pill in the pocket' not work. They know that should the rhythm not settle down quickly, they need to present to hospital for review.

within 48 hours, electrical

The other option, when a person presents to an accident and emergency department, is the use of electrical current over the heart to restart the heart or shock it back into normal rhythm. This is **D**irect **C**urrent cardio**R**eversion, DCR. It uses 'paddles' and requires a light general anaesthetic. It is very quick and generally very effective.

within 48 hours, my practice

In general terms, if a relatively well patient without structural heart disease or a history of heart problems presents with a new onset of atrial fibrillation, my normal practice is to put that person on anticoagulation immediately, often using one of the new novel oral anticoagulants as they are extremely effective.

I then ensure the patient has some heart rate control to improve the symptoms. I tend to use a reasonable dose of digoxin given intravenously in an attempt to achieve heart rate control as soon as possible.

I also give the patient some beta blockade as, very often, this may help return the patient to normal rhythm. With all that adrenaline pulsing through the patient because of the fear associated with the episode, it will dampen down some of the sympathetic drive.

Lastly, I sometimes use flecainide through the vein as an infusion over 30 minutes so that, if the heart returns to normal rhythm during the infusion, I have the opportunity to turn off the medication.

beyond 48 hours

If the patient has been in atrial fibrillation longer than 24-48 hours, we have crossed a threshold. The chance of a clot, or thrombus, forming in the left atrial appendage is too high to proceed directly to electrical or pharmacological cardioreversion, even with subsequent anticoagulant cover. In this situation we delay restoration of sinus rhythm until after three-to-four weeks of full anticoagulation.

beyond 48 hours, my practice

My preference is to wait a minimum of four weeks to give the body the best chance to clear, or break down, any possible clot that may be lurking in the left atrial appendage. I bring the patient back for review and check the ECG to assess rhythm. Sometimes the patient has reverted on the medications used to control rate. If that has happened, great, although the patient runs the unavoidable situation of the heart returning to normal rhythm while there is possibly a clot in the left atrium.

Should the patient still be in atrial fibrillation at four weeks, if the heart has a relatively normal structure and the patient is still troubled symptomatically, I will generally consider **electrical cardioreversion** as a planned procedure. This is a common procedure and relatively safe.

Before cardioreversion we look into the left atrial appendage to check there is no visible clot. This is done using a special ultrasound probe that goes down the patient's gullet so that we can look from very close range, as the oesophagus rests adjacent to the left atrium at the level of the diaphragm. This gives us the chance to actually see into the left atrial appendage which is not possible using a standard echocardiogram which is done through the chest wall.

We call this special ultrasound a **Trans** (through) **O**esophageal (gullet tube) **E**chocardiogram or TOE[15]. So, if the person is still in atrial fibrillation after four weeks and restoration of normal rhythm is indicated, we will proceed to a TOE DCR[16].

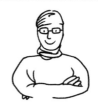

Often when I tell patients the next step is to slide a tube down their throat, have a close look at the heart, then, if all is OK, pull the tube out and give them a whack with electricity, they seem concerned. It sounds worse than it really is, although it is not without risk.

I explain they will have a light general anaesthetic for the entire procedure, so there will be no awareness of the TOE probe or the 'whack' of the DCR. I also make it really clear that we are doing the procedure because, based on the heart structure, there is a reasonable chance of success. I underline that we are undertaking this procedure to return them to normal rhythm, to make them feel better as the atrial fibrillation is causing unacceptable symptoms.

In explaining the risks involved, I try to ensure that patients understand that the risk of the procedure is outweighed by the benefit. I quote a complication rate of approximately 1-in-5000 of major complication with the TOE, a complication rate of approximately 1-in-10,000 for the DCR and a rate of 1-in-10-to-15,000 for the general anaesthetic. Although these risks are small, they are real. And it is not an exercise to be undertaken repeatedly without significant consideration of the pros and cons.

The need for repeated TOE DCR may be the start of the conversation about progressing to an **electrophysiological ablation** of the atrial fibrillation, or perhaps accepting permanent atrial fibrillation.

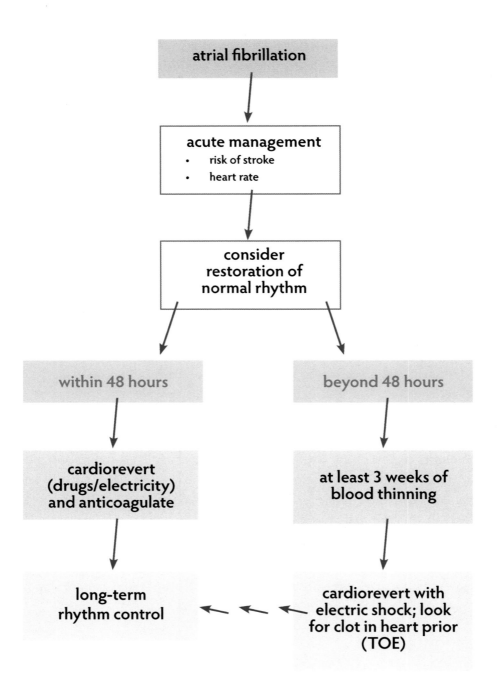

returning the heart to normal rhythm

dilated right atrium

When I met him, Jeff was 46 years old. He had just completed a 1/2 marathon, a 1/2 marathon running uphill and in good time! After the event he developed atrial fibrillation and ended up in the accident and emergency department with an irregular pulse.

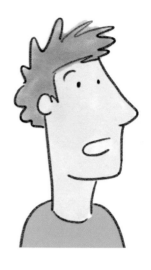

When I saw him in A&E, the ECG was normal. We anticoagulated him, slowing his heart down with digoxin, immediately. Because his heart was structurally sound, based on his exercise capacity, I also gave him flecainide to try to revert the heart: 150 mg intravenously, as an infusion over 30 minutes. That didn't revert him. Twelve hours later, I repeated the flecainide but this time gave him only 100 mg. This worked. He returned to sinus rhythm and he felt considerably better. We sent him home soon afterwards. He had anticoagulant tapering for the next couple of days and we followed him up in clinic.

The follow-up was interesting because when we looked at his Holter monitor he was getting extra beats from the top of his heart. We call these atrial extras (extras, extra beats) or supraventricular (supra, above; ventricular, main pumping chamber) atrial ectopic beats or atrial ectopics (ectopic, out of place). We also did an ultrasound of his heart to look at its structure and function. Interestingly, the right atrium appeared to be dilated; the left appeared normal. I had been expecting to see a normal-looking heart and I wasn't really sure what to make of this subtle and unexpected finding.

Jeff was in and out of hospital several times during the next year or so, with episodes of atrial fibrillation that were months apart and which responded reasonably well to therapy in the accident and emergency department.

Initially, we tried him on beta-blocker. He didn't tolerate that particularly well and I was comfortable switching him over to calcium channel blocker which can sometimes be slightly more effective in the setting of atrial ectopic beats.

I was, however, intrigued by the increase in the size of the right atrium. This was unusual and I wondered if it could be contributing to his low atrial fibrillation threshold. I ordered imaging of the connections of his heart, using cardiac CT imaging, so we could see how the great vessels interrelated with each other. As suspected, this showed an abnormality. It showed that two of the right upper lobe pulmonary veins drained directly into the right atrium. This meant that blood which should have been draining into the left atrium, then ventricle and then around the body, was draining instead into the wrong side of the heart, so that the right atrium was receiving blood, not only from the body but also from the lungs. This increase in blood flow caused an increase in volume and that increase in volume had stretched the right atrium. This was the cause of the anatomical observation of his right atrium being dilated. I believe this was a contributory factor in his development of atrial fibrillation in an otherwise structurally normal heart, in an otherwise well patient, without any other clear-cut risks.

Currently, Jeff is on a good dose of the calcium channel blocker, verapamil. I also have him on a blood pressure-lowering agent, the angiotensin-converting-enzyme (ACE) inhibitor, perindopril, as this may help with the remodelling of the chambers of the heart.

I am pleased to say that Jeff is well and stable. He carries with him a 'pill in the pocket' regime so that if he does develop atrial fibrillation, he is able to take extra verapamil and can start an anticoagulant to immediately reduce the risk of stroke. Of course, he is instructed to present as soon as possible after an event so that it might be dealt with appropriately.

He is having perhaps one, maybe two, episodes of atrial fibrillation a year. Although we have spoken about the possibility of using electrophysiological ablation to try to reduce the risk of recurrence, the frequency is not sufficient to justify that procedure at this stage.

Jeff is going well. I think he has an interesting, likely contributing factor in his development of atrial fibrillation. We catch up on a regular basis for on-going re-evaluation of the management plan that is now in place.

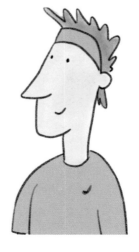

- Returning a patient to sinus rhythm has symptomatic benefits; surprisingly it does not reduce the risk of an adverse event in the long term.

- Sinus rhythm is restored by drugs or electrcity.

- Treatment needs to look at rhythm control as well as anticoagulation and is dependent on
    - the timing of presentation in relation to the episode
    - the structure of the patient's heart
    - the general medical condition of the patient.

- Over time, patients become used to living with AF.

---

[15]   in the USA, TEE, Trans (through) Esophageal (gullet tube) Echocardiogram

[16]   in the USA, TEE DCR

How does a patient stay in normal rhythm?

Chapter 8 -
How does a patient
STAY IN NORMAL RHYTHM?

Once a person has been returned to sinus rhythm, can efforts be made to keep the person 'on track' in normal rhythm, remembering that currently atrial fibrillation can't be cured?

The short answer is, "Yes".

However, there are several factors that drive our decision:

- unacceptable symptoms,

- age (the younger the person is the more likelihood of success), and

- the structure of the heart, in particular the left atrium.

There are also a number of considerations that need to be kept in mind when making the decision:

1) We want to keep people in normal rhythm to reduce symptom load so that they feel better.

2) We understand that our rhythm control treatments are moderately effective most of the time, but we rarely have a perfect result.

3) We accept that, as there is no cure, we are looking to reduce the rate of recurrence and the time people are in atrial fibrillation.

4) If we are dealing with one agent, then it is possible that we may need to add in another therapy or we may need to swap therapies to achieve some reduction in the time the person is in atrial fibrillation.

5) Our medications can generate rhythms of their own (be proarrhythmic) and this can be a problem.

6) We need, always, to try to ensure that we are balancing therapy safety with effectiveness.

With this in mind then, what are the steps we can undertake to try to maintain sinus rhythm in a person who has atrial fibrillation?

reversible factors

The first important thing to do is to address the reversible factors.

If the patient is significantly **overweight,** we want to improve that immediately. We know that weight has an impact on the way atrial fibrillation will recur. Very importantly, weight also has a very big impact on **obstructive sleep apnoea** or paused breathing while asleep at night. If obstructive sleep apnoea is present this needs to be addressed as the heart comes under a significant load if oxygen is not getting around the body properly.

If **alcohol** is central to triggering atrial fibrillation, we would encourage the patient to understand how alcohol intake can impact on the recurrence of AF. We would also check **blood pressure** and **thyroid function** and, encourage the patient to **exercise** and to manage **diabetes** or other medical conditions.

medications

Having addressed these reversible lifestyle factors, we then consider medications.

My practice is to use **beta-blockers** as a first-line therapy. These are broadly available and, on the whole, they seem to be well-tolerated for their effectiveness. A number of guidelines do not necessarily support the use of beta-blockers for maintaining sinus rhythm but, clinically, I repeatedly see patients who achieve long, symptom-free periods while using beta blockade. They are relatively safe, and my clinical experience suggests they are effective in a wide range of people, particularly those whose atrial fibrillation can be brought on by emotional triggers.

For those people for whom beta-blockers are not ideal, I will often use a **calcium channel blocker,** particularly in patients whose ECG monitoring shows extra atrial beats. For some reason, they seem to respond very well to **verapamil**. Again, current guidelines do not necessarily support this as a therapy for the maintenance of sinus rhythm. However, I observe that these agents can be beneficial for certain individuals. I know cardiologist colleagues who have had similar experiences.

If beta-blockers and calcium channel blockers are not working, or are not particularly well-tolerated, I might prescribe **flecainide.** Generally, I will use flecainide with a little bit of beta blockade, hoping for some effectiveness from both agents without pushing either agent too hard. Keeping doses as low as possible can reduce the possibility of side-effects while receiving benefit from two agents with two different actions.

If I use flecainide without a beta-blocker or without a calcium channel blocker, I will often use it with a small amount of **digoxin.** This is because we know that flecainide can increase the conduction of electricity through the AV node[17] which may increase the rate responsiveness of the atrial fibrillation for the individual should that person go back into AF.

Agents such as **amiodarone, dronedarone** and **sotalol** can also be used. They are more powerful agents, the next step up. These agents need to be closely monitored and regular ECGs are an important part of management.

electrophysiological ablation

Lastly, in very specific cases, for example for younger patients who

- are quite symptomatic with atrial fibrillation,

- have a fairly normal looking heart, structurally,

- fail control on a beta-blocker and, say, flecainide, or

- are now progressing to using a next line agent such as amiodarone or sotalol in the longer term,

I would next consider an **ablation** of atrial fibrillation using **electrophysiological technologies.** This modifies the atria in such a way that we alter the threshold of atrial fibrillation. My experience is that it is a really good way of achieving ongoing management and maintenance of sinus rhythm in the longer term.

It is really important, however, to understand that EP ablation is not a cure, nor is it for everyone. Used for the right patient, AF is less likely to redevelop quickly and it can provide up to several years of symptom-free sinus rhythm. I tend to combine it with a small dose of the beta-blocker or calcium channel blocker.

what is electrophysiological ablation?

Electrophysiological ablation is another method used to restore and maintain sinus rhythm. Electrophysiological simply means pertaining to the electrical function of the heart; ablation means destruction or removal.

Highly-trained cardiology specialists, electrophysiologists, who have a very detailed understanding of the electrics of the heart, perform the procedure.

As we have seen, electrophysiological ablation becomes a possible treatment when lifestyle modifications, together with a drug regime, do not effectively control symptomatic AF.

There are muscle cells that make up the left atrium called atrial myocytes. It would seem that protrusions of these myocytes can be found in the pulmonary veins as a consequence of embryological development during the formation of the atrium while in the womb. The problem is that these extensions of muscle cells into the vein are not meant to be there. As these cells are out of their usual location, in the veins, they are not subject to the same regulatory factors. This means that they can fire off intermittently and create a disturbance within the electrical milieu of the left atrium, thus creating a focus for the development of atrial fibrillation.

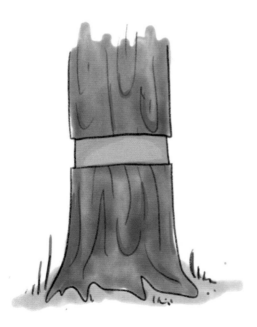

Electrophysiological ablation separates those cells in the veins from the cells within the left atrium.

Imagine one of the pulmonary veins coming into the left atrium. We 'ring-bark' it, literally separating the cells within the pulmonary vein which may be exciting the cells in the left atrium causing erratic and chaotic activity.

This 'ring-barking' is called **pulmonary vein isolation.**

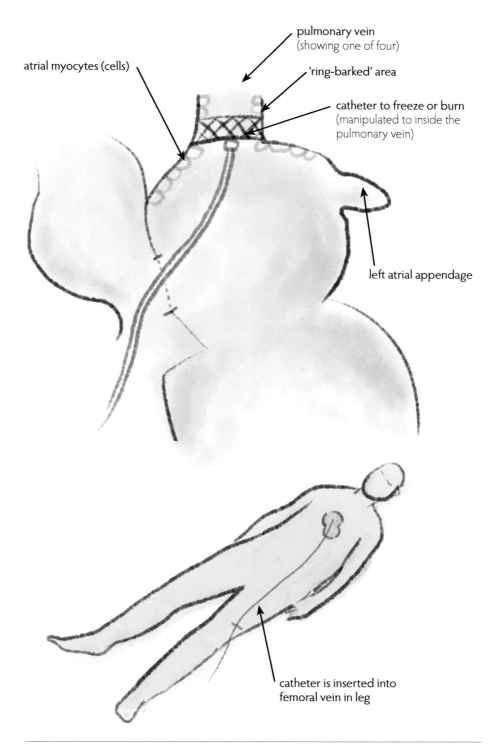

pulmonary vein
(showing one of four)

'ring-barked' area

atrial myocytes (cells)

catheter to freeze or burn
(manipulated to inside the
pulmonary vein)

left atrial appendage

catheter is inserted into
femoral vein in leg

EP 'ring-barking' of pulmonary vein

There are increasingly more clever techniques becoming available but essentially pulmonary vein isolation is a catheter technique. A long tube, or catheter, is used, along with radiofrequency, freezing or burning techniques, to damage the pulmonary vein tissue in a ring-like formation. The resultant scarring separates the misbehaving cells in the vein from the cells that are in the left atrium, leaving these cells, hopefully, to move together in an orchestrated way.

Of my patients, about 70 to 80 percent have a very successful result so that in the long-term they do well. Maybe five to 10 percent of patients will require a repeat procedure. Who goes for a second visit, the time frame and in what circumstances, are dependent on the patient's specific situation and the experience of the doctor. The person's symptoms must be weighed against the risk of the procedure and the risk associated with the underlying condition.

Electrophysiological ablation is a tremendous technology.

We tend to use it only for patients who are younger and/or who are symptomatic of atrial fibrillation, as well as those whose hearts are relatively structurally sound. If the heart is significantly unsound structurally, the chance of success is markedly reduced.

As with every procedure, there are risks. Major complications of EP ablation are quoted at between 1-in-5000 to 1-in-10,000. So this is an important conversation to have with your doctor to ensure it is right for you.

EP ABLATION PROCEDURE

The left atrium is quite deep in the body. The proceduralist generally gains access to the venous system in the leg and then passes a special catheter up to the right side of the heart. That catheter will cross between the atria, through the atrial septum from the right side to the left side and then, by rather impressive manipulation, the catheter is placed into each of the four pulmonary veins. A circumferential derangement of the cells, burning or freezing, or ablation, is performed. The procedure can take several hours.

The electrophysiologist has some tools for guidance. A CT scan of the left atrium gives a visual of exactly the shape and placement of those pulmonary veins. Generally, the patient will be on an anticoagulant at that time because if we are deranging those cells we are creating 'rough spots' in the veins, and those 'rough spots' could be a focus for the formation of a clot.

Although it sounds complicated, the patient often leaves hospital the day after the procedure. Its specialist nature, however, means that it is not performed in all cardiac units. For example, patients in Tasmania where I practise currently travel to Melbourne to have the procedure.

athlete who progresses to EP ablation

When I first met him, Tony was a very fit and very active 58-year-old man who had spent his life in the pursuit of fitness. He was an endurance athlete, a very high-level swimmer, runner, cyclist and a rower. He had participated at the top levels of his sports for many years. He still trained every day, often for several different events. Tony had quite a lot of stress at work and was having a difficult time with 'restructuring'.

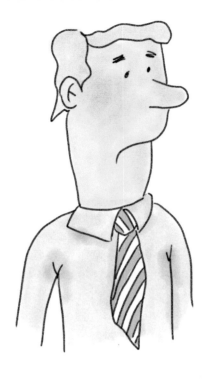

I first saw him a number of years ago when he was having episodes of atrial fibrillation between six and 12 months apart. When there was more stress at work, his atrial fibrillation was more frequent. This is a recurring story, not just for Tony.

With regard to the management of his overt, paroxysmal atrial fibrillation, when we looked at his predicted risk of stroke based on his CHA2DS2-VASc score, he scored zero, which is a low risk. This measurement considers cardiac failure, hypertension, age, diabetes and other factors that could increase a person's risk of an AF-related stroke. As Tony's score was zero and his symptoms waxed and waned with changes with his work, I put him on low dose aspirin. I also prescribed him a 'pill in the pocket' which was a number of tablets that he could take when an episode occurred so that his heart would slow, giving it a chance to return to normal rhythm. It worked well for him.

Over the next year or two, the work situation settled, and his atrial fibrillation episodes became less frequent.

Several years later, however, having established an alternate career, and with all things going well in his life, Tony presented with the recurrence of episodes of atrial fibrillation. This time, the occurrences were more frequent, more intense and clearly interrupting his daily living, particularly his exercise. These episodes were not related to stress. They represented the progression to an increased propensity to develop atrial fibrillation with time and age.

A decision was taken that he should have an EP ablation of his atrial fibrillation, to maintain normal rhythm. Using special catheters placed in the heart, a highly-trained specialist in a major hospital performed a pulmonary vein isolation procedure, a way to 'ablate' atrial fibrillation. This went very well.

Since then, he's been essentially free of atrial fibrillation.

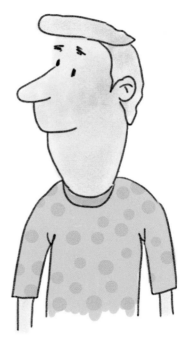

We chose that particular approach because he had had intolerances or difficulties with different drugs and as an athlete, he was keen to remain drug free if possible.

Although Tony presented some challenges to management, he is doing well. His work situation is good and, for the moment, his atrial fibrillation is only a memory. I keep an eye on him because we know there is a reasonable chance that, as he ages, the condition will return. For the moment, though, it's a matter of time and a matter of surveillance.

CAN I USE SUPPLEMENTS OR COMPLEMENTARY PRACTICES?

SUPPLEMENTS

Many of my patients are interested in using supplements. Is this wise?

When it comes to atrial fibrillation, there is not much data available. Some studies have looked at magnesium and others at fish oil in the setting of post-operative cardiac surgery and found no benefit.

Having said that, I do not have a problem with my patients using **magnesium** *as it seems to dampen atrial and ventricular ectopic beats for some and has also been shown to help keep blood pressure down.*

Fish oil *is fairly commonly used for joints and general health. Currently, there are no good studies to suggest it has an impact on AF. However, research tells us that omega 3 oils can stabilise the membrane of heart cells, so it should help.*

Can fish oil help reduce heart attacks and death?

Although the fairly recently released ASCEND[18] trial suggested, in a fairly low risk group of individuals, that fish oil made no difference, there have been a number of studies that suggest it is beneficial. These include the recently published REDUCE-IT[19] trial in which good doses of fish oil were given to high risk patients who had high triglyceride levels. Chat with your doctor about this situation.

Does fish oil increase bleeding?

In my hospital, many of the surgeons caution their patients not to take fish oil before surgery, although for doses of up to three or four grams per day studies have not shown any increase in the risk of bleeding or an impact on bleeding even if on warfarin. However, if my surgeon asked me to stop a supplement before surgery, I'd take the advice.

For daily living, I am happy with my patients eating oily fish or taking fish oil. I take some fish oil daily and eat oily fish once a week for my joints, with the feeling that it is probably a good thing for my heart.

As for any other supplements, I tell my patients to check with someone who has expertise and experience using supplements to ensure that they are not taking something that may interfere with their mainstream medications.

Remember if you are supplementing with a vitamin K preparation, it will interact with warfarin.

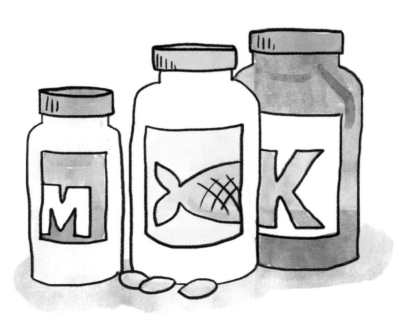

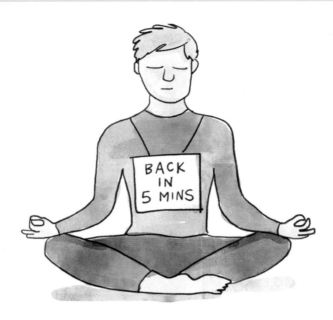

COMPLEMENTARY PRACTICES

Exercise regularly. Modest regular exercise will alter cardiovascular risk and with that, the likelihood of developing AF. So, please, try to keep active.

An interesting study has been undertaken by the University of Kansas Hospital. The researchers investigated the impact of yoga on atrial fibrillation[20]. They took a group of patients and followed them for three months as a baseline, and then started a twice weekly yoga regime with home practice. Comparing the before and after, yoga reduced the rates of AF by nearly 40 percent. Isn't that fantastic!

So, if you have AF, don't be surprised if your doctor tells you to take a deep breath and relax. Your medical practitioner is quoting evidenced-based medicine.

- Although there is no cure for atrial fibrillation, some patients can be kept in sinus rhythm for years.

- Factors contributing to the decision to keep the patient in normal rhythm include
  - the unacceptable nature of the symptoms
  - the age of the person
  - the soundness of the heart's structure.

- Keeping a person in sinus rhythm is achieved by
  - addressing reversible factors such as weight, obstructive sleep apnoea, alcohol consumption, high blood pressure,   thyroid function and control of other diseases
  - medication
  - EP ablation.

---

[17]   Remember, that special electrical conductor between the atria and the ventricles.

[18]   ASCEND (A Study of Cardiovascular Events iN Diabetes) New England Journal of Medicine 2018; 379:1529-1539

[19]   REDUCE-IT (Cardiovascular Risk Reduction Icosapent Ethyl for Hypertriglyceridemia) N Engl J Med 2019; 380:11-22

[20]   University of Kansas Hospital (the impact of yoga on AF trial) Journal of the American College of Cardiology 2013 Mar 19; 61 (11): 1177-82

What about the situation that is a bit tricky?

Chapter 9 -
How do we DEAL WITH COMPLICATED SITUATIONS?

As we routinely look to anticoagulate patients to reduce the risk of clot formation in the heart and a subsequent stroke, this makes anticoagulation a really important component of our management. Yet ...

what if we are dealing with a patient who is **elderly, frail and liable to fall?**

This is a complicated issue which I have covered to some degree with the HAS-BLED score, the score which assists with attempting to determine the risk of bleeding. However, in general terms, the clinician, with the patient, in an open and frank discussion, will need to try to ascertain the patient's ability to deal with anticoagulation, including the patient's risk of falling, hitting his/her head and bleeding. We need to be very specific, engaging the patient in a discussion about how the patient believes he/she will cope with those risks on a daily basis. In general, the doctor will wish to see the patient on blood thinning because, as I say to my own patients, "It is easier to deal with a bleed than a stroke" (the exception of course being a bleed in the brain, but this is less likely).

I've had elderly patients who remain active and are not frail. I had one patient who regularly went into the bush where he used a chainsaw. He had been a logger all his life and that was not going to change. So, we took this into account when deciding on his care: the man being 80+ years of age, in the bush with a chainsaw and other sharp pieces of equipment, and a long, long way from help. He still went on anticoagulation, but not before a detailed discussion which led him to understand the pros and cons of his situation.

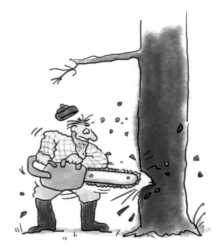

So, a case of the elderly and/or the frail, who are likely to fall, may well be when the clinician and the patient need to discuss what would work best, perhaps reducing doses, perhaps using alternate agents and certainly weighing the risk-benefit.

who has need of **a stent in a narrowed artery?**

Narrowed arteries and atrial fibrillation can be common bed fellows.

The incidence of both can increase with age, and some of the risk factors, such as hypertension, are also common. So, it is no surprise that sometimes a patient with atrial fibrillation also has a narrowed artery that needs to be opened.

One way is to open the artery by using a stent. A stent is a fine metal scaffold that is inserted into a narrowing in an artery and then is expanded to keep the artery open.

It is a great technology when used in the right situation and it is a terrific technique to enable the blood to flow more freely again. There is a catch, though, and the catch is that the metal of the stent is seen as a foreign material by the platelets.

When platelets encounter foreign material, they interpret that as a cut in a blood vessel and go to work forming a clot to heal it. **Problem!** We don't want a clot in an artery as the clot will block it. **Bad news!**

In regular situations, the way to overcome the clotting is to give the patient drugs that prevent the platelets from clumping. Such drugs are called antiplatelet agents. Aspirin is the most well-known.

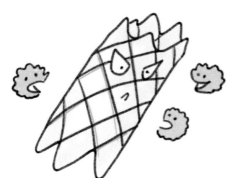

However, and importantly, in the setting of stenting, two antiplatelet agents or **D**ual **A**nti**P**latelet **T**herapy (DAPT) are needed to prevent clot formation.

problems with a stent: platelets want to stick to it

Most often patients will remain on DAPT for a minimum of three months to a maximum of 12 months. During this time, as DAPT is preventing clot formation, the inner layer of the blood vessel grows over the metal struts of the stent, thus preventing the platelets from interacting with the metal.

This process starts immediately. By **one month** the process will have produced reasonable coverage, by **three months**, a pretty good coverage and by **12 months** the stent, generally, will be completely covered.

What if the patient has atrial fibrillation and is already on an anticoagulant? Does the patient then take a blood thinner and two antiplatelet agents?

Think about the high risk of a bleeding complication that scenario may carry: medication to block the coagulation cascade **and** two medications blocking platelet function.

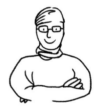

This situation needs to be dealt with using caution and care.

*Remember, **antiplatelet agents** are not effective for the clot forming in the left atrial appendage, while **anticoagulants** are not effective for clots forming on stents. So, a patient in AF with a new stent needs DAPT and anticoagulation to protect the stent and reduce the risk of AF-clot formation.*

Generally, the objective is to minimise any risk of a clot forming in the stent, while offsetting that against the risk of the patient having a problematic bleed.

As the highest risk of stent thrombosis is in the first 30 days, patients will be on two antiplatelet agents as well their regular anticoagulant.

Depending on the complexity of the stent and other patient-specific issues, this triple therapy will be stopped after the first 30 days or continued for about three months when one antiplatelet will be stopped. One antiplatelet and the anticoagulant will be used until month 12.

At 12 months, generally, the antiplatelet agent will be stopped and the anticoagulant continued long-term.

Guidelines related to these decisions are available and your cardiologist will be the most up to date with current practice should you be in this situation.

who has **cardiac failure?**

Cardiac failure brings to light another group of patients in whom AF has been shown to worsen prognosis.

If possible, we like to see patients in cardiac failure brought back to normal sinus rhythm as they have better outcomes. This is the case whether it is cardiac failure due to a poor functioning ventricle or cardiac failure in which the ventricle appears to contract 'normally'.

A relatively recent trial called CASTLE-AF[21] showed certain patients definitely did better if they could be maintained in sinus rhythm. Of course, in AF they also run a much higher risk of stroke.

So, if the patient is also affected with cardiac failure, the clinician will try to keep the patient in sinus rhythm, understanding that if there is **any** chance of the person being in atrial fibrillation, the person really does need to be anticoagulated to reduce the very high risk of stroke complications.

who has **severe renal failure?**

Renal failure is one of the situations where atrial fibrillation can be more prevalent. As patients with renal failure have a greater risk of bleeding, we need to be very careful.

Chronic end stage renal failure patients in atrial fibrillation are most likely to be managed with warfarin. This needs regular monitoring and levels can fluctuate depending on external variants.

We know also that NOACs generally need at least some renal function to be cleared from the body. If they accumulate, complications may arise. The NOACs are not ideal, then, for the patient with advanced renal failure. There are clear guidelines available to help doctors know the cut off points for renal function that are acceptable for prescription of the NOACs.

However, in cases where mild or moderate renal failure is present, there is very good data to support the use of NOACs as an alternative to warfarin, as long as the renal function is sufficient to allow adequate clearance of those drugs from the patient's system, and so remain safe.

who has **other complications?**

complication: AV malformations

I have a patient, Betty, who developed atrial fibrillation in her late 70s. That's not uncommon but the difficulty in Betty's situation was that I had been monitoring her for the previous 10 years, or maybe more, for a leaky mitral valve which had required surgical repair. As a mitral valve leaks, blood regurgitates into the left atrium leading to left atrial stretch. This had happened over the years before her surgery. Until the development of her atrial fibrillation, it had not been a significant problem. We were tracking the functioning of the valve and she had been on a low dose of aspirin in relation to her valve repair, blood pressure and some known coronary irregularities.

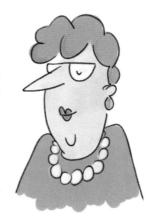

*The other concern with Betty, however, was that she had a very difficult condition to sort out: bleeding from her small bowel. It is called an **ArterioVenous** malformation or an AV malformation. This is a vessel abnormality which can bleed, unpredictably, spontaneously and significantly. Betty had had these AV malformations over a number of years.*

So, here is a patient

- *on low-dose aspirin for mitral valve repair, hypertension on treatment and minor coronary artery irregularities on treatment;*

- *with a history of mitral regurgitation which is going to drive atrial fibrillation because of left atrial stretch, and*

- *who also has a condition that leads to unpredictable bleeding.*

Tricky!

With her development of atrial fibrillation, we took a considerable time trying to use medications to keep her in sinus rhythm. This worked initially.

However, her atrial fibrillation progressed, albeit intermittently, to a point where we needed to look at reducing her risk of stroke.

I elected to use a NOAC and specifically one known to have a reversal agent, or antidote, readily available. This means that if she presents at the local hospital with a significant bleed from her AV malformation, there is a reversal agent available that could stop that bleeding almost immediately.

Betty carries the risk of a stroke but there is also a real risk of her bleeding from her gut. Both are catastrophic. I'm running her on a low dose of NOAC and, to-date, all is going well for her.

complication: cerebral bleed

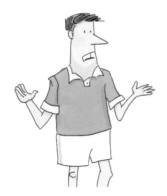

Tom is in his mid-to-late 70s. He had atrial fibrillation and he was appropriately managed on warfarin in the pre-NOAC era.

Unfortunately, the INR, or coagulation, caused by the warfarin increased and Tom had a cerebral bleed; his blood was thin enough that it bled into his brain. This caused a substantial stroke. He remained in atrial fibrillation but, for a time, the doctors caring for him did not want to give him an anticoagulant again because of the history of bleeding into his brain.

When I saw him several years after the haemorrhagic stroke, I said that his ongoing risk was probably greater from the formation of a clot within his heart and subsequent stroke than another haemorrhagic stroke. This risk could be reduced if we used one of the newer NOACs which would have a better anticoagulant control and without the fluctuations that can be associated with warfarin. So, Tom started on a dose of one of the NOACs.

Several years later, thankfully, there have been no troubles. We have reduced the risk of a thromboembolic stroke, or a clot from the heart going to the brain, and there have been no further haemorrhagic strokes or 'bleeds'.

complication: pre-excitation syndrome

Another difficult situation I would like to discuss is a condition called a pre-excitation syndrome.

In a normal heartbeat the electrical signals from the atria pass through the AV node into the ventricles. In a few patients, there is a connection directly between the top of the heart and the bottom of the heart which is a muscular band or bridge. This is in addition to the AV node. Now, as we know, the importance of the AV node is that it slows down electrical activity from the top of the heart to the bottom of the heart; it acts as a capacitor.

In a normal heart, when the patient goes into atrial fibrillation not all the chaotic electrical activity is transmitted to the lower part of the heart because the AV node slows down some of the chaos; it protects the ventricles. In the setting of this extra pathway, there is no slowing down the electrical activity; there is no filter; there is no capacitor.

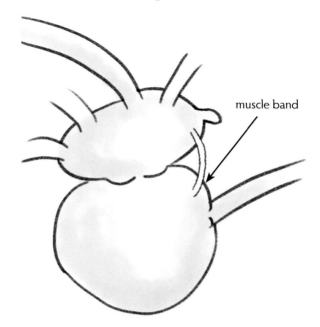

muscle band

In a patient with this direct connection between the atrium and the ventricle, a setting called pre-excitation, the chaotic electrical activity of atrial fibrillation is transmitted directly down that muscular band to the ventricle. This could lead to a very fast heartbeat or, at worst, ventricular fibrillation which means death.

A pre-excitation syndrome is also called Wolf-Parkinson-White Syndrome named after the people who first described it.

A pre-excitation pathway is a very difficult thing to deal with in the setting of acute atrial fibrillation.

In the short term, one wants to stabilise the atria as best as possible.

Most drugs used in AF management slow down the AV node, the normal conduction pathway. Those drugs are contraindicated if a patient has atrial fibrillation **and** a pre-excitation syndrome because the normal pathway is slowed down but the abnormal pathway is preferentially advantaged. So, drugs such as digoxin, metoprolol and calcium channel blockers often cannot be used in that setting.

If an agent is selected, it is a bridging strategy. In that situation, an agent such as amiodarone might be appropriate.

My experience is that the safest treatment, however, is to immediately use electrical current to revert the patient. More often than not, the person's condition is quite unstable.

The longer-term objective is to have this patient considered for destruction of the abnormal pathway using electrophysiological ablation techniques, a process of tissue injury similar to that used in an EP ablation of AF. That patient may also be considered for an atrial fibrillation ablation at the same time. While the individual is having the abnormal pre-excitation connection ablated, it is a great opportunity to isolate the pulmonary veins to reduce future occurance of atrial fibrillation.

Wolf-Parkinson-White Syndrome combined with atrial fibrillation is a very complicated situation. Clinicians will understand the risks it carries.

complications: lifestyle challenges, hypertropic cardiomyopathy

We met in 2003. Bob was 42 years old and weighed 140 kg. He suffered from obstructive sleep apnoea and was intermittently using a Continuous Positive Airways Pressure (CPAP) machine which forces air into the lungs during sleep to keep the oxygen levels up. His blood pressure was 160 to 170 over 90 (elevated).

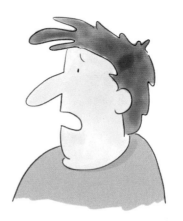

He came to see me because of an abnormal ECG which we evaluated with stress testing. We found no problems with the way his heart worked but certainly there were changes on the ECG that were not within the normal range.

At the time, I talked to him about the value of trying to reduce his weight. Over the following year he dropped approximately 25 kg in weight and felt better for it.

A visit in 2004 was the last time I saw him until 2012.

By 2012, he had developed atrial fibrillation. Given that blood pressure, obstructive sleep apnoea and weight are all significant contributors to the condition, it was no surprise. Initially, the atrial fibrillation was relatively well-controlled on medication and he was having episodes intermittently. He still had the same changes on his ECG, which we describe as deep T wave inversion. Basically, it was a change in the way the heart re-polarised and it didn't look normal. I was concerned about that.

Between 2003 and 2012, available technology had changed, so I ordered a cardiac CT scan which allowed us to have a really thorough look at the arteries of the heart. The advantage of a CT scan is that it also gives us very clear imaging of the chambers of the heart which we can then slice in 90° planes or orthogonal views. This just means we can get great views of the heart and can literally pick it up and move it around as we want, using our sophisticated work stations with their high-end graphics.

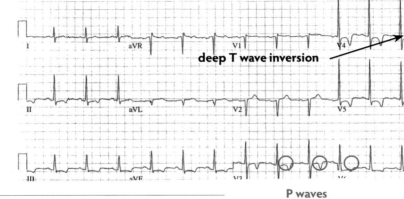

deep T wave inversion

P waves

Bob's ECG before the development of AF

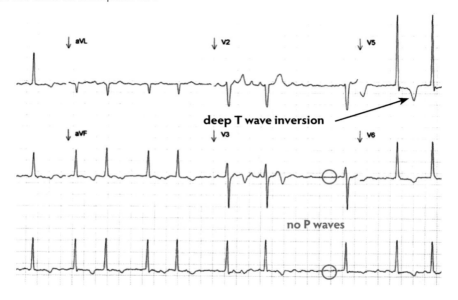

deep T wave inversion

no P waves

Bob's ECG after the development of AF:
the P wave is gone and the beat is 'irregularly irregular'

By doing this I was able to clearly demonstrate a couple of really important findings. Firstly, that Bob had a considerable build-up of plaque in his arteries. Secondly, I also made the diagnosis of a condition called hypertrophic cardiomyopathy *(hyper, increased; trophic, growth; cardio, pertaining to the heart; myopathy, a muscle condition or an increase growth of heart muscle problem).* **Hypertrophic cardiomyopathy** *is a thickening of the wall of the main pumping chamber of the heart, a thickening of the wall of the left ventricle. As it has a strong genetic link, it is important to screen in families.*

This is not a good thing for the heart.

A thickened muscle may not relax as well as normal muscle and so this condition can lead to increased pressures within the left ventricle. Those pressures are transmitted back into the left atrium with the consequence of stretching or dilating that atrium in the longer term. Remember, a big left atrium is a marker of future atrial fibrillation.

Hypertrophic cardiomyopathy is a significant contributor to the possible development of atrial fibrillation.

So, on top of weight, blood pressure and sleep apnoea, Bob had hypertrophic cardiomyopathy, a stiff heart, contributing to the likelihood of the development of atrial fibrillation.

In 2012, Bob again engaged in weight loss because he had regained most of the weight he had shed previously. He was able to lose about 20 kg.

In 2013, he was in and out of AF and was quite symptomatic with it. Part of the reason was the hypertrophic cardiomyopathy. The benefit of a properly contracting left atrium is that the left ventricle fills better, allowing the heart to work more efficiently. Once you take regular, left atrial contractions away, the heart needs to rely on passive filling or, simply, the flow back to the heart. With thickening of the muscle, the stretch of the left ventricle may not be as good as normal and pressures can build up so that the patient becomes quite symptomatic.

In 2013, there were a number of episodes when we cardioreverted Bob because of his symptoms. Although he successfully embraced weight loss, he was still a big man at well over 100 kg. With that being the case, and wanting to maintain sinus rhythm, principally because of his symptoms, I sent him for electrophysiological assessment and consideration of radiofrequency ablation of atrial fibrillation.

Initially he had good results from this but when the atrial fibrillation came back, we added extra therapies. One of these recommended by the electrophysiologist was the medication, amiodarone. One of the issues with amiodarone is the amount of iodine it contains. That high content of iodine means that it can interact with the thyroid gland. It will affect about 25 percent of patients.

After using it for several months, it did start to affect Bob's thyroid gland. Although amiodarone had been working well in controlling his atrial fibrillation, we had to stop it because of the impact it had on his thyroid function.

Some six months after his first EP ablation, towards the end of 2013, he was still having recurrent atrial fibrillation. The electrophysiologist suggested a repeat EP ablation. This second ablation was more successful than the first. Bob was able to remain symptomatically well-controlled in sinus rhythm for most of the next two years.

In the second half of 2015, however, he re-presented; back to his morbid weight, his blood pressure was still elevated, and he was using the CPAP machine for his obstructive sleep apnoea. His left atrium had dilated gradually over the years, due in large degree to the hypertension but also to the hypertrophic cardiomyopathy. He was also symptomatic again. Although we spoke again about the possibility of repeat electrophysiology ablation, I thought two attempts in the face of his other medical issues were as much as we could offer. As Bob was keen to explore further, he visited the electrophysiologist again, only to receive similar information as I had given him. The electrophysiologist reassured Bob that not much ground would be gained by trying again to retain sinus rhythm for him in the long-term.

We are now several years past 2015. As I have observed in many other people, over the course of a year or so the symptomatic effect of atrial fibrillation, as long as it is well controlled in terms of the heart rate, is often accommodated by the individual. Although it takes a while, the patient generally becomes used to it.

Now, Bob's heart rate is under control. He is anticoagulated. He is on good blood pressure control. He is on a cholesterol-lowering agent because the CT scan demonstrated significant plaque. We are trying to engage him in lifestyle modification, continuing with weight loss and exercise as much as possible. Symptomatically, he is as good as we can hope for and he even enjoys a round of golf once or twice a week. We've also taken the opportunity to screen his family for the condition that led to the thickening of his left ventricle, the hypertrophic cardiomyopathy.

Bob's is a complicated case and one that represents some of the many challenges associated with atrial fibrillation.

- There can be significant individual complications to take into consideration when managing atrial fibrillation. Each patient needs to be treated in relation to his/her particular circumstances. Rarely is AF treatment 'off the rack'.

[21] *CASTLE-AF trial (Catheter Ablation for Atrial Fibrillation with Heart Failure)* New England Journal of Medicine *2018; 378:417-427*

Conversations I often have ...

HOW
CONVERSATIONS

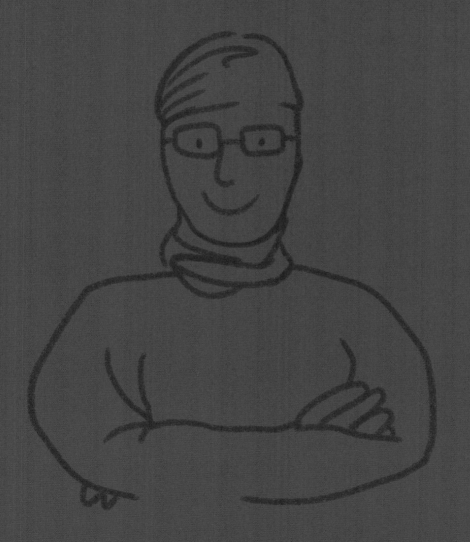

Chapter 10 -
CONVERSATIONS I HAVE WITH MY PATIENTS

reversing the effects of warfarin and NOACs

It is wonderful that we have such a range of anticoagulation medication available. However, there are times when the effect of that medication needs to be reversed, often quickly. This can happen, for example, in an emergency setting if a patient has a broken leg, is bleeding internally or needs urgent surgery.

There are two main groups of anticoagulants currently in use in Australia: warfarin and the named **N**on-vitamin K **O**ral **A**nti**C**oagulants) or NOACs.

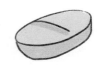

Warfarin is a drug that works through the vitamin K dependent factors of the coagulation cascade and the NOACs work at precise locations within the coagulation cascade. *(Please see page 84.)*

When it comes to reversing anticoagulation, the simplest way to achieve it is to withhold the anticoagulation medication. With time, the body produces the factors involved in the coagulation cascade and the system returns to normal. However, for most agents, this will take several days.

In the emergency setting, there is a need to reverse the anticoagulation quickly. This is particularly so in the case of severe haemorrhage when, regardless of the anticoagulant that is being used, fresh frozen blood products are 'poured' into the patient.

This literally replenishes the clotting factors that have been blocked by the anticoagulant, quickly returning the coagulation, or clotting, system back to normal.

These blood products are the products collected during donation of blood at blood banks. They are scarce, valuable and expensive resources.

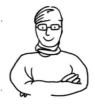

Some of my patients say they would prefer to stay on warfarin and use vitamin K as an 'antidote'. They have heard or been told by well-intentioned, but misinformed, parties that vitamin K is the antidote for warfarin. The reality is that the vitamin K-dependent factors take time to produce. So, if a patient on warfarin has bleeding problems and is given vitamin K to overcome the blocking effects in a bid to restore the coagulation system, the liver needs to produce those factors to have the system working again.

It can take six hours or more for the vitamin K-dependent cofactors to start being produced. In the acute, very urgent setting of severe haemorrhage, that process is not fast enough. In that setting, and other urgent scenarios, blood products need to be injected into the person to do the job quickly enough.

In the case of the NOACs, one of the agents, dabigatran, has an antidote that, when injected into the body, binds with dabigatran and makes it inactive. Called idarucizumab, it works almost immediately and is an ideal solution in the setting of uncontrolled bleeding.

Two other NOACs, apixaban and rivaroxaban, have an antidote, andexanet alfa, under development. The trials look promising. If it becomes available, which seems likely, it, too, will be injected into the patient to restore the coagulation system very rapidly.

Access to idarucizumab, and andexanet alfa (if or when it becomes available to clinical practice) means that bleeding patients on a NOAC will not need plasma products 'poured' into them if they are having an emergency bleeding problem. Instead, they will simply receive the appropriate antidote to reverse the action of the blood thinner.

....

Pretty good, eh?

....

Should I swap warfarin for NOACs?

Current guidelines suggest that if an anticoagulant is to be started for a patient with new atrial fibrillation then a NOAC is preferred, understanding that it is not the case if the patient has a mechanical heart valve or mitral stenosis. Similarly, if there are troubles stabilising an INR, warfarin can be swapped to a NOAC.

However, what if the patient is already on warfarin and stable? Patients often wonder if they should or could be on one of the newer anticoagulant agents.

Current wisdom suggests "if it ain't broke, don't fix it", but is there any data to help us?

A paper which pooled the data of more than 40,000 AF patients on either warfarin or a NOAC showed that the rate of stroke was lower in patients taking the NOAC.

In fact, it was nearly 20 percent less and the majority of that difference was driven by a reduction of bleeding into the brain, or haemorrhagic stroke. Surprisingly, this was the case even if the INRs were considered well controlled.

This meant that, overall, the patients taking a NOAC had a lower mortality rate of approximately 10 percent. The NOACs did, however, demonstrate an increase in gastrointestinal bleeds, a somewhat unpalatable problem, but better than bleeding into the brain!

So, what does one do?

While there is no trial looking at this question specifically, nor do current guidelines have a position on changing, my suggestion is to speak with your doctor about the pros and cons for your particular situation.

Having said that, I think if I had AF and was on warfarin, I would be looking to swap to one of the newer agents.

They are easier, with no regular testing needed; they appear safer than and as equally effective as warfarin, and if a NOAC with a single daily dose is chosen, then they are also convenient. Remember, however, there are specific criteria to be met for them to be prescribed and funded in Australia.

Tachycardia Polyuria Syndrome

Interestingly, over the years, I've had a number of patients describe very clearly that they need to go to the toilet to pass urine when a rhythm disturbance manifests itself. This is called tachycardia polyuria syndrome or fast heart (tachycardia), leading to an increase in the production of urine (polyuria). Its first documentation was in the 1960s.

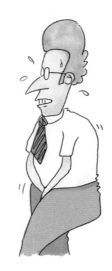

Tachycardia polyuria syndrome tends to occur when the patient is in normal, or sinus, rhythm for most of the time but experiences intermittent episodes of the fast arrhythmia. Usually the heart has been beating at more than 100 bpm for at least 20 minutes before the syndrome occurs. More often than not, the palpitation will arise and then 20 to 60 minutes later the need to pass urine follows. This need to pass urine can last for one or two hours, or even up to eight hours, but it depends on how long the rhythm disturbance lasts.

Why does this occur?

We believe that there is a change in pressure in the atria. In atrial fibrillation, as the chamber is not working properly, blood that keeps coming in from the veins and is not pumped out properly can then pool and stretch the atria. This muscle stretch causes a release of special proteins, or messengers, from the atrial tissues into the circulation. These messengers are called atrial (coming from the atrium) natriuretic (producing urine) peptides (mini proteins). So, the stretch on the top chambers of the heart from this arrhythmic disturbance gives rise to the production of messenger peptides which go to the kidneys and tell them to let more fluid go, or release urine.

This syndrome can occur in different types of rhythms within the atria, such as atrial fibrillation or flutter and re-entrant (a short circuit loop) supraventricular tachycardia. It also seems to be different in different people.

It is an interesting scenario and one that I see occasionally. It is not a condition that needs treatment of its own, as treatment of the underlying rhythm will prevent the syndrome occurring.

Do I need a pacemaker?

I am frequently asked by patients with atrial fibrillation if they need a pacemaker. The general answer is "No".

A pacemaker is a device to provide electrical impetus for the heart when the heart is not producing enough electrical stimulation itself. So, pacemakers are a solution to the heart beating too slowly.

If we think about what is happening in atrial fibrillation, the top part of the heart is beating too quickly, in fact, chaotically. That activity is bombarding the AV node with electrical impulses and those impulses are driving the ventricle to rapid contraction, the 'irregularly irregular' heartbeat of atrial fibrillation. So, in general terms, atrial fibrillation does not need a pacemaker because the heart is not going slowly; it is going too fast. Atrial fibrillation generally needs heart rate regulation that slows the heartbeat down, **not** speeds it up.

Easy? Well, things are never that simple.

Occasionally, as is always the case, there are exceptions.

While trying to control the rate of AF, sometimes the medications may not be well tolerated, or they don't work very well. In these occasional situations, we consider isolating the atria from the ventricles altogether. We do that by AV electrophysiological ablation, a procedure in which we use special catheter techniques to ablate the electrical connection completely, between the top and the bottom of the heart.

This means that the heart, left to its own devices, would generate a heart rate commensurate with what the ventricle would generate by itself, and that is too slow. So, when we do an AV nodal ablation for atrial fibrillation we also insert a pacemaker to ensure that the heart rate is maintained.

There are also situations in which the electrical systems of the heart can be affected by a degenerative process that leads to the failure of the AV node, leading to a 'heart block'. This condition, just like the deliberate AV nodal ablation, separates the atria and ventricles electrically and will need a pacemaker to maintain an adequate heart rate. This is not linked to the presence of AF and its occurrence represents a second process in the patient, although the frequency of both increases with age.

Do I need a stress test or angiogram?

This is a question that is commonly confronted. It is important as atrial fibrillation and coronary artery disease[22] are common companions.

In general terms, if a patient presents in atrial fibrillation with a rapid heart rate, faster than for the expected maximum for that age, then the heart has been put through an auto 'stress test'[23]. If at a fast heart rate there are no chest pains and no features on the ECG[24] to suggest a lack of blood flow to the heart, then it is likely there are no major blockages in the major arteries.

One confounder is that often when a 'cardiac patient' presents at a hospital, a blood test for troponin is performed. This is a really useful test when a patient presents with chest pain.

It returns a positive result when there has been significant strain on the heart. If it rises over time, it could point to possible narrowing of the arteries. If it does not rise, then the heart is less likely to have been the cause of the pain, although it cannot be excluded.

An arrhythmia such as atrial fibrillation can increase the troponin, so how is this dealt with?

My practice is to consider the management based on the presentation:

- ***rapid atrial fibrillation, no chest pain, no ECG changes and no troponin rise***

It is hard to make a case for a stress test or an angiogram in this setting, so I treat the atrial fibrillation as appropriate. Later, a more thorough assessment of cardiovascular (CV) disease risk can be made, including absolute risk assessment, plus perhaps the use of imaging. Early use of an invasive angiogram in this setting, 'just to be sure', is more than over-cautious; it is probably over-servicing.

- ***rapid atrial fibrillation, with chest pain OR suggestive ECG changes OR positive troponin***

In this scenario, there may well be an issue with the arteries. The use of risk-modifying drugs becomes important in association with a plan to further evaluate and assess the coronary arteries. My practice is to investigate using an invasive angiogram in highly suggestive situations. I would likely use a stress test or cardiac CT imaging in an intermediate risk patient.

- ***rate-controlled or asymptomatic atrial fibrillation***

I treat the atrial fibrillation and then work through the process of CV risk assessment.

Can I be screened for AF?

We know a significant percentage of patients have no symptoms and so will be 'under the radar'. Research is telling us that with one-off rhythm screening in the community of otherwise well individuals over 65 years of age, atrial fibrillation is detected in 1.4 percent. This is about what we would guess from prevalence figures. If we were to provide a hand-held device to 75 year olds for them to check their rhythm twice a day for two weeks, we would likely detect atrial fibrillation at a rate of three percent. These pick-up rates could be increased if we were to screen people who already have increased CHAD scores, meaning the higher-risk population.

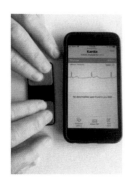

At this stage it seems that opportunistic screening, meaning when the individual perhaps sees the local doctor, rather than systematic population based screening is more cost effective. However, the technologies are changing constantly and the goal posts are likely to shift.

There are devices that link to a smart phone and provide a rhythm trace. New smart phone-compatible watches are even being equipped with a rhythm sensing feature.

As amazing as this seems, remember that these personal devices, at least in the early stages, are most likely to be used by younger members of the population who may not be the ones most at risk. Perhaps grandchildren can check out their grandparents?

Also, these devices are likely to over-interpret the presence of atrial fibrillation. As we know not all irregular rhythms are AF, so could these devices 'over call' it, thus burdening the health system or creating unnecessary stress for the individual? Time will tell.

Although this is not dedicated screening, the regular interrogation of implanted devices such as pacemakers and loop recorders can demonstrate presence of AF. You might also like to check your pulse occasionally.

Do I need to store AF drugs is a particular way?

Dabigatran should be kept in its original packaging until the time it is taken. Do not put the capsules in a pill box or organiser unless it remains in its foil wrapper. There are no specific storage requirements for warfarin, apixaban and rivaroxaban, beyond keeping them in a cool dry place that is secured and away from children.

How often do I need testing or to see my cardiologist?

The answer to this question will vary depending on your response to treatment although, generally, your cardiologist will see you more often at the beginning of your AF management, and then see you less frequently as the situation becomes more stable.

I see patients a few weeks after an initial diagnosis of atrial fibrillation to ensure that they have remained well and are tolerating the medications. Then I start to stretch out the visits.

If patients are on flecainide, I will see them between six and 12 monthly to repeat an ECG, as the width of the QRS complex can be a clue to the toxicity of the drug.

If they are on digoxin, I like patients to have their levels checked every six to 12 months. It is also important to check renal function. Worsening renal function can lead to digoxin and the NOACs being retained within the body, causing toxicity.

When checking a digoxin level it is generally required to be a 'trough' level, that is at its lowest level in the bloodstream, so the test should be taken just before the morning dose. I recommend that digoxin be taken in the morning so that the highest serum levels have the most effect on the patient during the activities of the day. Patients should hold their digoxin dose on the morning of the test and take it straight after the blood has been taken.

Remember, if the level starts to creep up, it may cause nausea and anorexia, so be aware of your last digoxin level if you go off your food.

item	test	frequency
warfarin	INR blood test	frequent until stable then 1 to 3 monthly
NOAC	no testing	watch renal function
digoxin	blood level test	6 - 12 monthly
flecainide	ECG	6 - 12 monthly
amiodarone	TSH blood test	6 monthly
heart rate	ECG or Holter monitor	6 - 12 monthly
heart function	echo (echocardiogram)	initially, then not needed routinely unless change in symptoms
coronary artery disease	stress test	not needed routinely unless change in symptoms

IMPORTANT POINTS   CONVERSATIONS WITH PATIENTS

- **reversing anticoagulation**
  - **non-urgent**, stop the use of agent and wait
  - **urgent**, vitamin K for warfarin reversal is **not** fast enough in an emergency
  - if there is **no reversal agent** available, then blood products are injected into patient to urgently provide clotting factors, regardless of anticoagulant used
  - dabigatran has a reversal agent that acts very quickly
  - apixaban and rivaroxaban are likely to have a reversal agent soon

- **swapping from warfarin to a NOAC**
  - a conversation should be had with your doctor

- **tachycardia polyuria syndrome**
  - a fast heartbeat can cause increased passing of urine for some patients

- **Do I need a pacemaker?**

(continued next page)

(continued)

- in most cases, no, but there are exceptions

- **Do I need a stress test or an angiogram?**
  - atrial fibrillation and coronary artery disease can be common companions; management is based on a patient's symptoms on presentation

- **Can I be screened for AF?**
  - yes; particularly recommended for people who are 65 years or older
  - checking one's pulse from time-to-time is worthwhile
  - changing technology is likely to change the goal posts

- **Do I need to store AF drugs is a particular way?**
  - storage: cool, dry and safe place
  - dabigatran must remain in foil until consumed

- **How often do I need testing or to see my cardiologist?**
  - this will depend on your response to treatment and the treatments on which you have been placed

---

[22]   Coronary artery disease or heart disease is the process of plaque build-up in the artery that leads to a narrowing of the artery and reduced blood flow that produces symptoms, such as angina, shortness of breath, heart attack.

[23]   Stress test is a functional test of the heart. It involves exercising the patient or giving the patient medication to replicate exercise to try to reproduce the symptom under investigation or unmask lack of blood flow to the heart.

[24]   An electrocardiogram shows the rhythm of the heart.

Another conversation I often have ... is with medical practitioners.

Chapter 11 -
CONVERSATIONS I HAVE WITH GENERAL PRACTITIONERS

a common phone call

Generally, people present with atrial fibrillation in one of three ways.

There are people who, when they develop atrial fibrillation and their symptoms manifest for the first time, go straight to **hospital** because the experience is new and it's scary.

There are others in whom the atrial fibrillation is found **incidentally.** For these people, there is generally not a sense of urgency as they feel well. Their situation needs to be addressed promptly so that the risk of stroke is reduced, and the heart rate is then evaluated and treated so it is well-controlled.

So, 'the phone call' I often receive represents the group in the middle.

People often walk into their **local practice** saying that they haven't been well for a few days. Maybe they have felt palpitations. Medically, they are relatively stable; they have not had a loss of consciousness; they have not had chest pain.

Such a scenario often elicits a telephone call from a general practitioner to me. The doctor wants to know whether or not this patient should be sent to accident and emergency immediately to have the possibility of atrial fibrillation treated. I always ask for a copy of the ECG to be sent through to me so that I can confirm the diagnosis, as occasionally, the problem may be an irregular pulse for reasons other than atrial fibrillation.

It is amazing how useful a smart phone picture and text can be.

My feeling is that if the patient is relatively stable and in reasonable health without any other associations that would raise concerns, we can manage this patient without an urgent visit to accident and emergency. It is relatively easy to find out about renal function, thyroid function and other co-morbidities.

I discuss with the doctor the important actions to be taken: reduce the risk of stroke and slow the heart rate. To slow the heart rate, I recommend digoxin therapy which can be given orally, and beta blockade, generally metoprolol, which also can be given orally. To address anticoagulation, the patient can start on a NOAC which will be simple to use, can be easily acquired with a script and its usage does not require monitoring.

I then suggest to the GP that I will follow up with that patient in the next week or two after we've had the chance to do some important testing. Particularly, I want to see the structure of the person's heart, using an echocardiogram.

I'll also make the point to the GP to tell the patient that should things not settle down, or should there be any trouble at all, to present immediately to accident and emergency.

If we are able to get some heart regulation started, together with some anticoagulation, generally we can stabilise this patient. Testing is done so that when I see this patient I have more information. Sometimes, we can even revert the patient to normal rhythm simply by these measures. And importantly, when I see the patient in my rooms, if there is the decision for direct current cardioreversion, we are almost halfway through the three to four weeks of anticoagulation needed before attempting such a procedure.

For a reasonable number of patients, we can be methodical, institute appropriate therapy, avoid an unnecessary presentation to accident and emergency, and effectively and efficiently manage the patient with available medications that can be given orally, gaining an excellent result for all concerned.

I'm always happy to speak with GPs who are unsure about how to proceed with the presenting patient. If I can help guide them through, of course, I'm happy to do that. Also, if there are any concerns, I will often have the patient come urgently to my rooms and we can take the treatment from there.

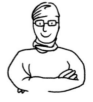

WHERE
THE FUTURE

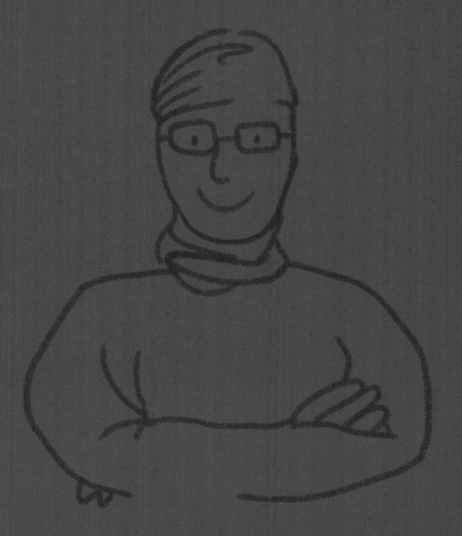

Chapter 12 -
LIVING WITH ATRIAL FIBRILLATION
globally and locally

Joe, patient, Hobart

When diagnosed, I was unaware that I had atrial fibrillation. I had been aware of 'something' but thought it was due to tension and pressure of work.

After being referred by my GP, we discovered that I was close to having a heart attack. This was something of a surprise as when I was younger, I had been fit, ate a healthy diet and there was no family history of heart problems.

After discovering the presence of atrial fibrillation, I soon began recognising the signs of an episode. Mostly, it occurred in the early hours of the morning when I was asleep. It would wake me up. I would feel uncomfortable, with a tightness in my neck, my chest pounding and sometimes with an ache in my arm. My brain felt as if it were scrambled; it was hard to think logically. When such an episode occurred, I would ensure I was warm and sit in a chair next to the phone until it passed. It was quite scary and at times I thought it might be the end.

I have had an ablation which worked for a time.

I also tried different medications and concentrations. Now the condition has settled down (except when I forget to take my medication). Even so, I often wonder when it will come back.

In the meantime, I am so thankful that with patience and trying different approaches. I am currently in a good position.

According to the European Society of Cardiology guidelines for the management of atrial fibrillation (2016), there have been major advancements in treatment and management strategies for atrial fibrillation in the past 20 years. As you have already read, oral anticoagulants and, in particular, more recently NOACs, have markedly reduced the incidence of stroke and mortality in atrial fibrillation patients. Other improvements, such as in rate control and rhythm control, have improved related symptoms. However, although they may have improved symptoms and cardiac function, reduction in long-term morbidity or mortality has not improved to the same extent.

The guidelines say that in contemporary, well-controlled and randomised clinical trials, the annual average stroke rate is about 1.5 percent and the annualised death rate is about three percent in anticoagulated atrial fibrillation patients. A minority of these deaths is related to stroke, while sudden cardiac death and death from progressive heart failure are more frequent.

Furthermore, atrial fibrillation is also associated with high rates of hospitalisation, commonly for management, but is often also linked to heart failure, myocardial infarction and treatment-associated complications.

Current figures for Australia, in terms of both prevalence and cost, are not available. Among the most recent publicly available are figures from a June 2010 report by Price Waterhouse Cooper[25]. This estimated that the annual costs to the Australian economy resulting from atrial fibrillation in 2008-09 were at least $1.25 billion per annum through medical costs, costs of long term care for those with a disability and lost productive output. By way of comparison, the cost per person with atrial fibrillation was more than double the estimated per person cost in relation to obesity and higher than the per person cost of cardiovascular disease or osteoarthritis.

Relying on international evidence to derive prevalence estimates for Australia, the report estimated that, in 2008-09, 240,000 people or 1.1 percent of the population suffered from atrial fibrillation, with more than half the sufferers aged over 75 years. It estimated that an extra 6300 people suffered a stroke for the first time as a result of atrial fibrillation and that there were 45,600 hospital separations for atrial fibrillation, more than for stroke or heart failure.

A 2011 Deloitte Access Economics report, *Off beat: atrial fibrillation and the cost of preventable strokes,* uses an atrial fibrillation prevalence rate of seven percent for people in Australia aged 50 years or older.

It estimated that nearly 62,000 strokes would occur in Australia in 2011, including 45,873 first-ever strokes. Nearly one-third (14,364 of the 45,873 strokes) would occur in people with atrial fibrillation and three-quarters (10,709 strokes) could be specifically attributed to patients' atrial fibrillation rather than other clinical factors.

This is a serious condition with significant human and economic cost.

Although the figures quoted here might not be as recent as one would like, consensus in Australia and around the world says that both atrial fibrillation prevalence and cost are on a significantly rising trajectory.

If there is one thing that by now must be patently obvious, it is this. Atrial fibrillation comes in many guises and one treatment or management plan does not fit all. There is a compelling responsibility for individualising care that addresses not only patient treatment but the day-to-day management implications of living with atrial fibrillation.

CASE STUDY – LISA

pregnancy

Lisa was an otherwise well, slim and normotensive[26] 39-year-old mother of an 18-month daughter when she came to see me. Lisa and her husband were looking to have a second child as soon as possible as she was aware her biological time clock was ticking along. The problem was that Lisa had recently developed intermittent runs of atrial fibrillation which were escalating. There were some stresses at home and there were some stresses at work, and I'm not convinced these weren't contributing. However, there was no family history of atrial fibrillation, nor was there a history of alcohol.

At the time of reviewing Lisa, she was severely affected by the recurrence of atrial fibrillation almost every other day. It was interrupting her sleep; it was interrupting activities of daily living and was causing her a deal of panic and distress. An echocardiogram showed that she had normal heart structure and function. That, with a normal thyroid blood test, meant there was no clear-cut indicator as to why she had developed atrial fibrillation. Yet, she had.

I commenced her on a beta-blocker, metoprolol, and she responded well. However, for a woman who wanted to become pregnant, nurture a child through that pregnancy and then breastfeed the new baby, being on a beta-blocker, or any agent for that matter, was not desirable. I thought Lisa presented a situation in which it was paramount to try to control the atrial fibrillation as best as possible without medication, for the sake of a healthy pregnancy and the safe delivery of a child.

So, I discussed the situation with an electrophysiological colleague. I considered Lisa was a good candidate for electrophysiological ablation for her atrial fibrillation at the earliest opportunity. If successful, this could control the atrial fibrillation without therapy and allow a pregnancy, delivery and the early life of her new child to proceed without Lisa being on any drugs. My colleague agreed and was very helpful. We started medication for thinning the blood and we booked Lisa in for the procedure as soon as was feasible.

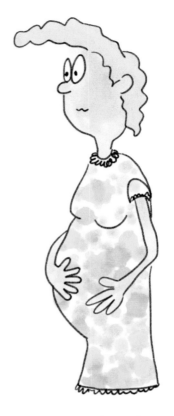

She had that done in six weeks. All went well. When I saw Lisa several weeks later, we stopped medications to see how she would react. I followed her up again in eight weeks with a clinical assessment. Up-to-date Holter monitoring showed no abnormality. The EP ablation had controlled her rhythm, she was feeling much better and looking forward to extending her family.

This was an unusual case. It was not what we would usually see but it was a situation in which the therapy was adjusted to suit the needs of the individual patient. I think this was a really good outcome. Lisa was happy and I'm waiting to hear about the new arrival!

I have been wondering if she has a boy if he might not be named after her cardiologist ☺

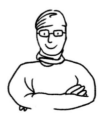

questions for daily living

For people who have atrial fibrillation, day-to-day living is often based around questions relating to very common issues, such as:

What effect does caffeine have in relation to AF?

Caffeine is a stimulant. It is also my preferred drug of addiction during the day. It commonly pops up in news articles as either 'good' or 'bad' for you. Probably, on balance, several cups a day will keep the world turning and is not a bad thing for your health. Over stimulation of the autonomic nervous system, however, can precipitate an event of atrial fibrillation.

I have patients who are clearly sensitive to caffeine and report the same. They cut back or avoid caffeine to help control their condition. Other patients don't seem as sensitive and continue to enjoy a cup or two a day without issues. It is case-by-case and individuals need to see how they respond. It is certainly a conversation to be had with your doctor.

Energy drinks with high levels of caffeine are probably best avoided.

Can I exercise safely?

Atrial fibrillation, of itself, is not a reason not to exercise. It is worth, however, noting a few things.

Firstly, when patients ask if they can exercise, they are really asking if they are going to have a heart attack, a lay term for a blocked artery.

Atrial fibrillation and blocked arteries are two different processes affecting the electrical system and the fuel lines, respectively. Although they are not linked directly, they can occur in the same individual. Both are common and the risk of each increases with the age of the person. Speak with your doctor.

Secondly, if you are in atrial fibrillation, is the heart rate well controlled? If it isn't, then exercising will only make the heart rate even higher and make exercise difficult.

Although, in general terms, we like to see our patients exercising, your best course of action is to check with your doctor to ensure that he or she is happy with your rate-controlling medications and the possibility of you exercising.

What if I need to have surgery?

In the past, if a patient on warfarin for atrial fibrillation needed to undergo a planned or an elective surgical procedure, then there was much fuss about managing the warfarin dosage around the time of surgery. Invariably, we would stop the warfarin about five days prior to the procedure and then put the patient on a 'bridging anticoagulation' regime that used injections of the blood thinner heparin, morning and night, until the day of the surgery.

This complexity is no longer necessary.

Recent research indicates, that in simple surgeries and where the AF is uncomplicated, it is safe to stop the warfarin before and restart it after the procedure. This is also the case with the newer NOAC agents. Missing these drugs for three full days prior to the procedure and for a few days after will suffice.

If the situation is more complicated, like a metallic valve replacement, a previous stent or by-pass grafting, cardiac failure, a complicated surgery, previous stroke or very large left atrium, then a plan needs to be put in place. Involve your cardiologist and ensure the plan is based on your risk of stroke and the risk of bleeding associated with your surgery. I like to see my patients who are in this situation so that I can ensure that nothing is missed and so that I can document that the patient has a good understanding of the risks and benefits. It can also be a timely catch-up and review.

Can I stop the medications if I feel well?

Taking tablets when feeling well is a real frustration for many patients.

However, remember, that in the context of atrial fibrillation, the medications will be keeping you in normal rhythm or controlling your heart rate, or reducing your risk of stroke. So, if you are feeling well, the medications are probably doing their job.

My strong recommendation is that if you have been put on medication, it is for a specific and good reason. Before unilaterally altering your management plan, it is best to speak with your treating doctor.

flexibility and juggling to suit the patient's need

Kevin is a 79-year-old man (2018) whom I met for the first time about eight years ago when he had an episode of atrial fibrillation. He had had AF previously and I met him in the setting of an intermittent episode.

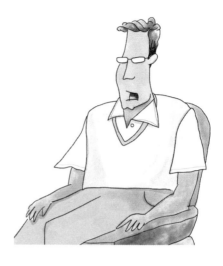

When I saw him the ultrasound of his heart was pretty normal, which was reassuring, although I did note that he was relatively anxious about the development of atrial fibrillation. It would also be fair to say, and Kevin wouldn't mind me mentioning it, that he was fairly sensitive to medication and he was very particular in his demeanour, at the more highly-strung end of the spectrum.

I increased his therapy. He was taking 80 mg of sotalol morning and night and I increased that to 120 mg of sotalol morning and night. I started him on warfarin to lower the risk of stroke and I sent him home.

Kevin was fairly stable for the next couple of years. I saw him again in 2014 when, every few months, he was developing short-lived paroxysmal (intermittent) atrial fibrillation. It seemed to coincide with times of stress or tension and it occurred predominantly at night. As he was relatively stable and protected by the anticoagulation, there was little else to do, although I did increase the sotalol to 160 mg morning and night.

In 2016, he was due for major surgery which carried with it a significant risk of bleeding. It was important at the time of the surgery that Kevin did not have any blood thinners in his system. The healing process which was to take several months also needed to be warfarin-free. So, when Kevin came to consult with me beforehand, my feeling was that we should add in another antiarrhythmic agent. I wanted to minimise, as best as possible, his episodes of atrial fibrillation while he was unable to take an anticoagulant. He was already on sotalol 160 mg morning and night. I elected to add in a small dose of flecainide, 50 mg morning and night, and stop the warfarin, as was required for the surgery.

My normal habit is not to combine sotalol, a class III antiarrhythmic agent, with flecainide, a class I antiarrhythmic agent, because of potential proarrhythmic effect, or causing rhythm problems rather than preventing them. However, I was keeping the flecainide level low and there was a very particular reason for doing it, the surgery. I also monitored him very closely with serial ECGs. One of the indicators that can give us a clue about toxicity developing through the use of flecainide is if the QRS complex on the ECG widens. A change in the Q-T interval can suggest sotalol toxicity. Both indicate that there is a change in the way the membrane of the cell depolarises. It is really important that we track these parameters.

Well, I'm pleased to say that when Kevin had the surgery, he didn't have a miss-beat. He was able to manage on both medications for two to three months without any atrial fibrillation of which he was aware. He was so pleased with the outcome he asked to remain on flecainide with the understanding that the combination of proarrhythmic agents could carry some risk. I was happy to oblige as long as he was happy for me to monitor him very closely.

Again, we checked his echocardiogram which demonstrated he had normal left ventricular function, normal heart structure and previous cardiac scanning had ascertained that he had no coronary artery disease. As his heart was structurally normal, the risks of a proarrhythmic problem were less than for someone who had abnormal function of the heart. We also knew that he had normal renal function, so it was unlikely that there would be an accumulation of antiarrhythmic agents.

Also, instead of reintroducing warfarin, I began him on one of the novel oral anticoagulants, rivaroxaban. This is working very well. He has been stable and happy with 'his AF' since.

One of the other aspects we need to look at closely in atrial fibrillation is blood pressure. As I continued to care for Kevin, it became apparent that his blood pressure was elevated and needed better control. Introducing new therapies was not that easy as he continued to be very sensitive to many medications. Calcium channel blockers, a common first-time blood pressure treatment, gave him headaches, while even a low dosage gave him swollen ankles.

After six to nine months of changing and altering his medications, we eventually came up with a very low dosage of the calcium channel blocker, amlodipine, on a daily basis, 2.5 mg per day. We used an agent called telmisartan at half the lowest dose tablet to be taken only on Saturdays, Sundays, Tuesdays and Thursdays. We also added in a medication called spironolactone, one tablet taken on Mondays, Wednesdays and Fridays. Eventually we had his blood pressure perfect. Unfortunately, it lasted only a couple of months when he came back to see me describing the side-effect of tenderness within the breast. This is a recognised side-effect of spironolactone. We swapped it with an agent that was very similar but less likely to have that side-effect in a male, the drug, eplerenone. Again, it was taken on Mondays, Wednesdays and Fridays. His blood pressure at the time of writing was perfect.

With this combination, Kevin was happy in terms of side-effects, while being well controlled in terms of his atrial fibrillation, blood pressure and his risk of stroke.

Why have I told you about Kevin? Sometimes we need to be flexible and patient as we seek to find what works for the individual, and that can take some juggling. As Kevin was cooperative in terms of trying to find what worked for him, we could work through the process in a systematic way. He remains well and very happy with his current care.

---

[25]   The Economic Cost of Atrial Fibrillation in Australia – *Price Waterhouse Cooper, June 2010*

[26]   *having a normal blood pressure*

Epilogue -
OVER TO YOU

By now you will understand that atrial fibrillation is a common medical condition, the symptoms of which can come and go, come and hang around for a while, or come and stay. In any scenario, once you have it, you have it for the remainder of your life. It cannot be cured, only managed.

Although its likelihood of occurring increases with a person's age, it can affect the young to the old, men and women, and more often than not comes when the body is under stress for other reasons; the very time you don't want an extra problem.

You can reduce your own atrial fibrillation risk by ensuring your blood pressure is well managed over your lifetime, maintaining a healthy weight which will also reduce your risk of obstructive sleep apnoea, and refraining from excess consumption of alcohol.

Don't be surprised when you develop AF if you are a snoring, overweight, committed imbiber with poorly controlled hypertension.

Most people feel the symptom of palpitation or notice a change in their physical capacity, yet not everyone knows that they have it. For some people, the first sign of the condition can be a collapse and for others it may be a stroke. In others, it may be discovered incidentally during another medical procedure.

For many sufferers, the symptoms can be debilitating, for others, they are an inconvenience. As your doctor, my aim is to minimise the symptoms as safely as possible and to maximise your prognosis. I want you to "live as well as possible, for as long as possible".

Medications and several procedures are available for treatment. Often, the more effective the drug, the greater its side-effects and one treatment does not fit all cases. Successful treatment is highly personalised and can take patience and perseverance to establish and maintain. In each case, the risk-benefit of any treatment needs serious discussion between the patient and the treating doctor.

Symptoms aside, the biggest concern regarding atrial fibrillation is risk of stroke, a catastrophic consequence that will occur on average at a rate of five percent a year in an untreated group of atrial fibrillation sufferers.

Blood thinners can reduce the risk of stroke by reducing the likelihood of the formation of a clot within the left atrial appendage of the heart. The blood thinners include good, old-fashioned warfarin which works by blocking vitamin K, and also the newer agents, the **N**on-vitamin-K-blocking **O**ral **A**nti**C**oagulants, NOACs.

People with atrial fibrillation need blood thinners, but people with AF also need operations and people with AF have accidents. Atrial fibrillation is a bleeding problem for those on blood thinners and a clotting problem for those not on thinners.

The risk of stroke must be balanced with the risk of bleeding, and both risks increase with age and the complexity of other medical conditions being suffered by the patient.

Development of the NOACs has been one of the single most significant advances in the management of atrial fibrillation in recent years as their ease of use provides much more convenient anticoagulation without the fluctuating dose adjustments and repeated blood tests needed with the use of warfarin, with the same or better efficacy.

If we look into a future that always holds promise, we can see electroporation, a new catheter ablation technology that can isolate culprit areas of the heart and pulmonary veins, without scarring. This will allow more extensive ablation therapies which should result in better outcomes.

Under development, also, is a system that uses 'proton cannons' to 'shoot' protons from **outside** the body into very specific locations within the heart to replicate the invasive catheter ablation techniques. Sounds amazing doesn't it?

There is also work going into the understanding of the 'brain' of the heart, the ganglia, the collections of nerve cells that form control centres adjacent to the atria. Current research is suggesting that these nerve centres have significant influence in the development of atrial fibrillation and that they may well prove a viable target for intervention.

However, until the future arrives, I strongly suggest now:

if you

- are already the 'proud owner' of AF, then visit your doctor for a thorough health check. Hypertension, diabetes, coronary disease and renal disease are common travelling companions of atrial fibrillation and these should be **properly evaluated and managed;**

- do not have atrial fibrillation, then see your doctor for a thorough health check. Hypertension, diabetes, coronary disease and renal disease are common travelling companions of atrial fibrillation and their **early control** could delay or prevent its onset, especially as you age;

- carry too much weight (you don't need your doctor to tell you, but you do need to find a reason to make a change), have a serious conversation with your loved ones and start to look after yourself;

- snore (your spouse has probably already told you), lose weight and if you still snore, see your doctor, as sleep apnoea is not good for you;

- drink more than two to three standard drinks a day (male) or more than two (female), it will catch up with you. Double the price of the wine you drink and halve what you consume. Alter your habits.

Daily, I see the suffering associated with heart disease and our specific interest here, atrial fibrillation.

Simple lifestyle maintenance can reduce your risks substantially. However, if you already have atrial fibrillation, attention to good management with the help of your medical practitioner can considerably improve your symptoms and so your daily living, for some, even providing lengthy symptom-free living.

My deep desire has been to provide you with information that can help you to be involved in your own destiny, to give yourself the best chance for a healthy life. It is now over to you. I wish you the very best.

Good health.

Dr Warrick Bishop
Hobart, Tasmania, Australia
April 2019

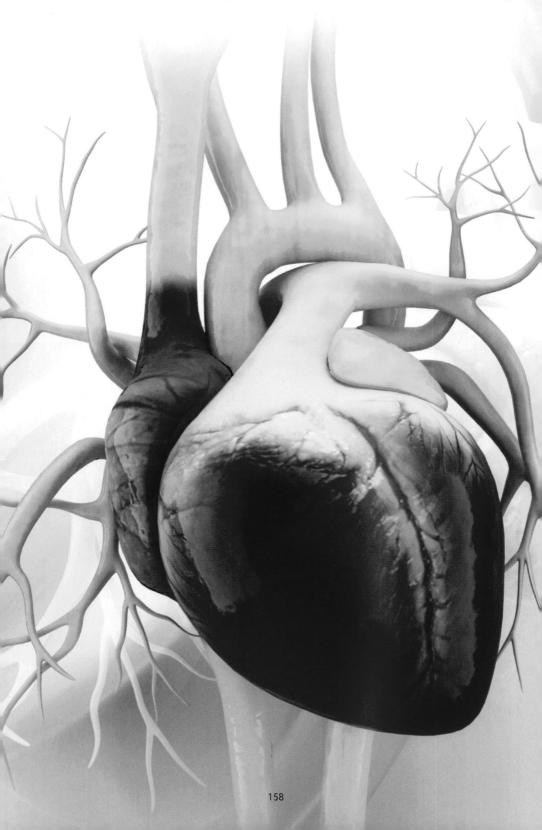

List of illustrations and tables

Glossary

Amiodarone

a powerful antiarrhythmic agent (returning the patient to, or keeping the patient in, normal rhythm); also useful in certain emergency situations for slowing the heart rate; long-term use for keeping the heart in sinus rhythm needs to be closely monitored

Angiogram

contrast (dye) injected into a patient that outlines the coronary arteries in exquisite detail, giving information about the location, the quality and nature of the plaque, the degree of stenosis and the size of the vessel affected. There are two types of coronary angiogram. One is often referred to as CT coronary angiogram or a CCTA, a coronary computed tomography angiogram. The other type of coronary angiogram is called 'invasive' and requires a small tube to be passed from an artery in the arm or leg to the heart to inject dye directly into the arteries.

Anticoagulation therapies

treatments to help stop a clot forming; keeping in mind the two major risks, the possibility of a stroke and the likelihood of bleeding

Apixaban

long-term blood-thinning NOAC that works through factor 10 in the coagulation cascade; has a reversal agent under development

Atrial fibrillation (AF)

an 'irregularly irregular' heartbeat characterised by the loss of the coordinated contraction of the top part of the heart, the atrial chambers, or atria. It affects the pumping capacity of the heart. The condition can be managed but not cured.

> **overt or symptomatic AF**
> the type the patient feels

> **silent or asymptomatic AF**
> the type the patient does not feel and is discovered as an accidental finding

> **paroxysmal AF**
> lasts between 24 and 48 hours but no longer than a week

> **persistent AF**
> lasts longer than seven days

> **permanent AF**
> is present for longer than a year

> **valvular AF**
> if the patient has a narrow mitral valve or artificial heart valve; is associated with a greater risk of a clot forming in the left atrial appendage

Arteries

the vessels of the body's circulation system that carry the blood away from the heart. The aorta, the biggest artery of the body, takes the blood from the left ventricle as the blood begins its journey around the body. The coronary arteries are the first branches in the body's circulation system.

> **carotid arteries**
> the major blood vessels to the brain

Associations

connected, joined or related

Aspirin

a well-known antiplatelet agent, used to help prevent blood clots

Asymptomatic

producing or showing no symptoms

Atrium

a pre-pumping chamber of the heart. There is an atrium on each side of the heart; the right atrium moves blood from the body through the right ventricle to the lungs, while the left atrium moves blood from the lungs through the left ventricle into the body.

Automaticity

an automatic depolarisation system of the cells of the heart

AV malformation

arteriovenous malformation is a malformation of the blood vessels; can produce unpredictable, spontaneous and significant bleeding

Beta-blockers

drugs frequently used to control the heart rate. They dampen the sympathetic nervous system which has nerve endings supplying the AV node, reducing the speed of electrical conduction from the atria to the ventricles and thus slowing the heart rate. Often used as a first-line therapy for keeping the heart in sinus rhythm, long-term. A commonly used agent is metoprolol.

Blood

the bodily fluid that conveys oxygen and nutrients to the body and removes carbon dioxide and other wastes. Among its components are platelets (which help in clot formation).

Blood clot (thrombus)

a soft thick lump

Calcium channel blockers

agents that affect the way calcium flows through the cell membrane, resulting in lower blood pressure and/or lower heart rate. Commonly used agents are verapamil, diltiazem, nifedipine and amlodipine.

Cardioreversion

medical procedure to bring the heart back to sinus rhythm using drugs or electricity

Causations

factors/actions that cause the problem

Clexane
injected drug for thinning the blood in an acute
setting; acts on factor 10 in the coagulation
cascade

Coagulation (clotting)
the process by which components of the blood
change from free proteins to a gel

Coagulation cascade
the process (a cascade of different factors)
by which a clot is formed. It has two key
components:

>**platelets**
>small cellular fragments that are
>important in the formation of clots

>**fibrin**
>a strong cross-bridging strand
>protein which forms the scaffold of
>the clot

**Coronary artery disease or
cardiovascular disease**
the process of atherosclerosis or plaque build-up
in the artery that leads to a narrowing of the
artery and reduced blood flow that produces
symptoms including angina, shortness of breath,
a heart attack

Dabigatran
long-term blood-thinning NOAC that works
through factor 2 in the coagulation cascade; has
a reversal agent

DAPT
dual **a**nti**p**latelet **t**herapy
two antiplatelet agents are needed to prevent
clot formation in the complicated situation of a
stent being needed to open a narrowing artery

DCR
direct **c**urrent cardio**r**eversion
use of electrical current over the heart to restart
or shock it back into normal rhythm; uses
'paddles' and requires a light general anaesthetic

Digoxin
a drug for slowing the heart rate by acting on the
AV node and thus slowing the ventricle

Diltiazem
a calcium channel blocker used to slow the
heart rate

Disease
a symptom or loss of normal function

Dronedarone
powerful antiarrhythmic drug used for
attempting to keep the heart in sinus rhythm
long-term; needs to be closely monitored

Echocardiogram (echo)
echo, sound, *cardio,* heart, *gram,* picture
a scan of the heart using ultrasound waves to
acquire a picture. It gives information about the
valves, the chambers of the heart and pressures
within the heart.

Electrocardiogram (ECG)

a trace of the electrical activity through the heart acquired by electrodes. It shows the rhythm of the heart. Features of an ECG can be used to determine the status of the heart muscle.

P wave

electrical activity in the atria, reflecting actual depolarisation or the electrical flow. No P wave with chaotic electrical activity is the diagnostic thumbprint of atrial fibrillation

QRS complex

created by the electrical impulses reflecting the depolarisation of the major muscle of the heart

T wave

the return of normal repolarisation to the heart muscle ready for the next beat

Electrophysiological ablation

specialist procedure which becomes a possible treatment when lifestyle modifications and drug regimes do not effectively control symptomatic atrial fibrillation

Flecainide

antiarrhythmic agent

Fibrinolytic system

factors that prevent a clot from extending too far

Heart

a large muscle that pumps blood through the body

Heparin

injected drug for thinning the blood in an acute setting; acts on factor 10 in the coagulation cascade

Holter monitor

a device worn by the patient for several days during normal activities as an aid to diagnosing atrial fibrillation

Hypertrophic cardiomyopathy

hyper, increased, *tropic,* growth, *cardio,* pertaining to the heart, *myopathy,* a muscle condition an increased growth of heart muscle or thickening of the wall of the left ventricle, the main pumping chamber of the heart. This condition is a significant contributor to the possible development of atrial fibrillation.

INR

International Normalised Ratio a worldwide standardised test for measuring a person's blood clotting speed to reflect warfarin levels

Left atrial appendage (LAA)

a recess within the left atrium where blood can pool when the atria are not functioning correctly (AF). A clot can form and subsequently dislodge, making its way to the brain where it becomes lodged in a blood vessel, leading to an ischaemic stroke.

Metoprolol
a commonly used beta-blocker, for heart rate control

Myocardium
myo, muscle, *cardium,* being of the heart
the muscle of the heart

NOAC
novel **o**ral **antic**oagulant or more recently named **n**on-vitamin K **o**ral **antic**oagulant; also known as DOAC or **d**irect **o**ral **antic**oagulant

now widely used for patients with non-valvular AF and who have adequate renal function, to reduce the risk of clot formation. Agents include apixaban, dabigatran and rivaroxaban.

Node

> **sinoatrial** (SA)
> is located in the top of the right atrium and it is where the electrical activity of the heart originates

> **atrioventricular** (AV)
> a cluster of cells in the centre of the heart between the atria and ventricles which allows electrical communication; also acts as a gatekeeper, regulating the electrical impulses as they enter the ventricles

Pacemaker
a device to provide electrical impetus for the heart

Palpitations
arrhythmic heartbeats

> *rapid and irregular*

> **atrial** (top of the heart)
> **ectopic** (out of place)
> **beats** (heartbeat)
> extra beats arising from the top part of the heart

> **ventricular ectopic beats**
> extra beats arising from the ventricular

> *rapid and regular*

> **atrial flutter**
> similar to atrial fibrillation except there is a re-entrant circuit occurring in the right atrium

> **supraventricular tachycardia**
> *supra,* above the ventricle,
> *tachy,* fast, *cardia,* pertaining to the heart
> an electrical short circuit in the atria that keeps firing on itself

> **ventricular tachycardia**
> a high-risk rhythm in the main pumping chamber of the heart

> **ventricular fibrillation**
> a cause of sudden cardiac death

'Pill in the pocket'
a pre-arranged, out-of-hospital, drug regime that can be taken by the patient immediately a problem arises

Pre-excitation setting
a muscular band which connects the atrium
and the ventricle (in addition to the AV node)
thus transmitting the chaotic electrical activity
of AF directly to the ventricle, bypassing the
gatekeeping of the AV node. Also known as
Wolf-Parkinson-White Syndrome.

Prognostic (prognosis)
improving the long-term outcome
for the patient

Pulse
the feeling under the skin from the contraction
of the left ventricle which makes the blood flow
through the body's arteries. This can be felt in
several locations including the wrist. In a healthy
heart, the pulse is strong and regular.

Reversal agent
a drug that can quickly stop the effects of
anticoagulation, especially useful in an
emergency situation that involves bleeding

Rivaroxaban
long-term blood-thinning NOAC that works
through factor 10 in the coagulation cascade; has
a reversal agent under development

Rhythm

sinus (normal)
the healthy heart rhythm, which is
controlled by the sinoatrial, or
sinus, node, beating in a
synchronistic and smooth manner

arrhythmia
when the synchronicity of the
heartbeat breaks down

Score

CHAD
cardiac failure, **h**igh blood pressure
(hypertension), increasing **a**ge and
diabetics
a clinical predictor for estimating the
risk of stroke in patients with AF

HAS-BLED
hypertension, **a**bnormal renal or
liver function, previous **s**troke,
previous **b**leeding problems
principally from the gut, **l**abile
control of warfarin (labile INR),
elderly (over 65 years of age), **d**rugs
or alcohol
a clinical predictor for determining
the risk of complications from
bleeding

Sotalol
powerful antiarrhythmic drug used for
attempting to keep the heart in sinus rhythm
long-term; needs to be closely monitored

Stenting

an intervention for coronary artery disease in which an intravascular device (balloon) within a wire scaffold is inserted percutaneously (through the skin) and guided to the site of the narrowing. When the balloon is inflated, the artery is opened. When the balloon is removed, the wire scaffold remains to keep it open. The scaffold is called

a stent.

Stress test

a test of heart function. It involves exercising the patient or giving the patient medication to replicate exercise, to try to reproduce the symptom under investigation or unmask lack of blood flow to the heart.

Stroke

a disruption of the blood supply to the brain leading to permanent loss of function

> **haemorrhagic**
> when a blood vessel ruptures and bleeds into the brain

> **ischaemic**
> when a clot (also called thrombus) blocks an artery, leading to a lack of blood flow. Such clots often form in the large blood vessels in the neck, the carotid arteries, or in the heart as a consequence of atrial fibrillation

> **TIA**
> *transient*, doesn't last very long *ischaemic*, lack of blood flow, **a**ttack a temporary disruption of the blood supply to the brain leading to loss of function, lasting less than 24 hours

Symptomatic improvement

improving how the patient feels

Tachycardia-induced cardiomyopathy

fast-heart-induced muscle problem; can be seen in patients who have silent, persistent atrial fibrillation

Tachycardia polyuria syndrome

tachycardia, fast heart, *polyuria,* leading to an increase in the production of urine

TOE

*t*rans, through, *o*esophageal, gullet tube, *e*chocardiogram an ultrasound probe that looks into the left atrial appendage to ensure there is no visible clot; often used prior to electrical cardioreversion

Troponin

a blood test used as a predictor when a person presents with chest pain to assess the likelihood of the heart being involved

Valve
(in order of blood flow)

tricuspid
a one-way valve between the right atrium and the right ventricle

pulmonary
a one-way valve between the right ventricle and the pulmonary circulation which takes the blood to the lungs

mitral
a one-way valve between the left atrium and the left ventricle

aortic
a one-way valve between the left ventricle and the aorta which is the main artery of the body

Veins
the vessels of the body's circulation system that carry the blood to the heart. The blood collects into two major veins, the superior vena cava and the inferior vena cava, before draining into the right atrium and then the right ventricle on its way to the lungs.

Ventricle
the main compression (pumping) chamber of the heart that pushes the blood through the body. There is a right and left ventricle. The right ventricle pumps the oxygen-poor blood to the lungs while the left ventricle pumps oxygen-rich blood into the body.

Verapamil
a calcium channel blocker used to slow the heart rate

Warfarin
a blood thinner used to reduce the risk of stroke. It blocks the vitamin K-dependant coagulation factors produced in the liver, factors 2, 7, 9 and 10.

Index

Thanks

Without help, encouragement and support from a number of people, this book would still be a good idea waiting to happen.

Colleagues whom I hold in the highest regard and who were generous enough to find precious time in their busy schedules to offer professional review and collegial encouragement included **Professor Garry Jennings AO** and **Dr David O'Donnell** who, of course, also provided the foreword and preface, respectively, and **Doctors John Saul, Michael McCarthy, Karam Kostner** and **Alistair Begg.** I would also like to acknowledge the contributors to the guideline papers that supported this book. The guideline documents are enormous undertakings driven by colleagues donating their time for better medical care.

I am grateful to **all my AF patients** who have contributed to my collective experience upon which I was able to base this book and especially to those whose stories are used throughout its pages.

Invaluable and frank patient-specific and man-in-the-street-comments were received from **Kelvin Aldred, Chris Bishop** (Dad) and the eagle-eyed, masters of detail **Rod Miller** and **David Thomas.**

And then there are technical professionals who also helped create this book. **Jillian Smith** brings precision and attention to detail in her editing and proofreading; designer and artist **Cathy McAuliffe** has an overflowing abundance of creative talent and **Penny Edman,** a writer who works with me, is the best, bringing focus, enthusiasm and passion.

To these collaborators in particular and to everyone else involved in the production of *Atrial Fibrillation Explained,* I am truly grateful.

About the authors

Warrick Bishop is a practising cardiologist with a passion for preventing cardiovascular disease. He has special interests in cardiac CT imaging, lipid management and eating guidelines.

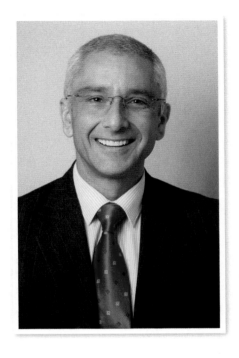

Warrick graduated from the University of Tasmania, School of Medicine, in 1988. He worked in the Northern Territory before commencing his specialist training in Adelaide, South Australia. He completed his advanced training in cardiology in Hobart, Tasmania, becoming a fellow of the Royal Australian College of Physicians in 1997. He has worked predominantly in private practice.

In 2009, Warrick undertook training in CT cardiac coronary angiography, becoming the first cardiologist in Tasmania with this specialist recognition. This area of imaging fits well with his interest in preventative cardiology and was the focus of his first book, *Have You Planned Your Heart Attack?* (2016). He holds level B certification with the Conjoint Committee for the Recognition of Training in CT Coronary Angiography and is a member of the Society of Cardiovascular Computed Tomography, Australian and New Zealand International Regional Committee (SCCT ANZ IRC).

Warrick is also a member of the Australian Atherosclerosis Society and a participant on the panel of 'interested parties' developing a model of care and a national registry for familial hypercholesterolaemia. He has also developed a particular interest in diabetic-related-risk of coronary artery disease, specifically related to eating guidelines and lipid profiles.

Warrick is an accredited examiner for the Royal Australian College of Physicians and is regularly involved with teaching medical students and junior doctors. He has worked with Hobart's Menzies Institute for Medical Research on projects in an affiliate capacity, and is recognised by the Medical School of the University of Tasmania with academic status.

He is also a member of the Clinical Issues Committee of the Australian Heart Foundation, providing input into issues of significance for the management of heart patients.

In addition to authoring the books, *Have You Planned Your Heart Attack?* and *Atrial Fibrillation Explained*, in 2018 he founded the Healthy Heart Network to further his reach in helping to prevent heart disease.

A keen surfer, he enjoys travel and music and playing the guitar with his children.

Penelope Edman is a freelance writer, editor and photographer based in Hobart, Tasmania, Australia. After beginning her print journalism career in Bundaberg, Queensland, in the late 1970s, she moved to Hobart in 1991. She is an Australasian award-winning journalist and editor, and her articles and photographs have been published throughout Australia and internationally. She authored four non-fiction books before assisting Dr Bishop with *Have You Planned Your Heart Attack?* and *Atrial Fibrillation Explained*.

Made in the USA
Columbia, SC
30 August 2020